LANGUAGE DEVELOPMENT AND ASSESSMENT

Studies in Developmental Paediatrics

Volume 1

LANGUAGE DEVELOPMENT AND ASSESSMENT

Joan Reynell

Formerly Senior Lecturer in Educational Psychology,
The Wolfson Centre, Institute of Child Health,
University of London

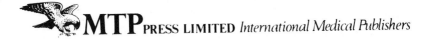
MTPPRESS LIMITED *International Medical Publishers*

Published by
MTP Press Limited
Falcon House
Lancaster, England

First published 1980

British Library Cataloguing in Publication Data
Reynell, Joan Katharine
    Language development and assessment. –
    (Studies in developmental paediatrics; vol. 1).
    1. Children – Language
    I. Title   II. Series
    401'.9   LB1139.L3

ISBN 0–85200–300–5

Text set in 11/13 pt VIP Palatino, printed and bound in Great Britain at The Pitman Press, Bath

CONTENTS

Contents

ACKNOWLEDGMENTS

Many people have contributed to the research on which this book is based. Space would not allow an individual mention of all these people, but I would particularly like to thank the following:

Professor Holt and the staff of The Wolfson Centre, Institute of Child Health, where most of the clinical research was carried out; Michael Curwen and the four speech therapists who helped with the revision of the Reynell Developmental Language Scales; Dr Jean Cooper and Mrs Molly Moodley, who combined with me in the research project reported in the last chapter; and again Dr Jean Cooper for reading and commenting on the script.

I am also grateful to the Editor of the *British Journal of Disorders of Communication* for permission to republish the data from the article which first appeared in that journal, reporting the findings from the five-year language intervention project.

I would also like to acknowledge, once again, the generous grant from the Department of Education and Science which made much of the work possible.

SERIES EDITOR'S NOTE

This is the first volume in a series of books entitled *Studies in Developmental Paediatrics*. This is a relatively new discipline which has attracted much interest and there is now a need for literature on the subject.

The practice of developmental paediatrics is not, however, confined to the 20th century. Several centuries B.C. Psamethicus is reputed to have reared two children apart in order to see whether they spontaneously developed speech. In France, in the 18th century, Victor, the wild boy of Aveyron was studied, after he had been captured in the woods, by Itard a young French doctor, who later developed educational methods for retarded and deaf children which were based upon his experiences with Victor. In England, in the 19th century, Charles Darwin, with his analytical mind, found delight in the scientific study of his own children. His findings are recorded in a book which was first published in 1872 and which is still available. It should be compulsory reading for all students of developmental paediatrics.

The turn of the century brought an intense activity in the field of child study. In Vienna, Freud taught that the child is father to the man. In France, Binet published intelligence tests the aim of which was to detect and assess handicaps early in childhood, so that the victims might benefit from special schooling. In America, Granville Hall, an admirer of Darwin, published work which encouraged interest in child psychology. What was probably the first infant welfare clinic was opened in 1896 by Witmer. It was realised that children are not miniature adults but human beings with structures and functions suited to their present state yet capable of development and that before maturity is reached each child will pass through many stages and phases of development.

The birth of modern developmental paediatrics, however, can properly be ascribed to Arnold Gesell and his co-workers. Working at Yale in the 1920s and 30s, he studied babies and children of all ages under many different situations and he was able to determine the developmental pattern of 'average' children. If the pattern taken by most babies is accepted as normal or 'average' then, Gesell argued, it should be possible to match a particular child against that pattern and estimate the present state of development. Because phases and stages of development follow in an orderly way – although the rate may vary – he further argued that some prediction is possible, as is a diagnosis of development.

Since Gesell's day, there had been an expansion of his work. Amatruda continued his work and Catell's tests and the Denver scales, both widely used in USA, are derived from Gesell's work. Ronald Illingworth, after studying with Gesell, worked in Sheffield and was a pioneer in England. He, in his turn, taught many of the present day developmental paediatricians, including Kenneth Holt, Britain's first professor of developmental paediatrics. There has also grown up what might be called the 'Guy's Hospital Group'. This was ably led by the late Ronald MacKeith. Peter Gardiner, one of the authors in this series, worked at Guy's, as did the late Mary Sheridan, who has been one of the most original thinkers and whose tests of hearing and vision are now part of our heritage. There have been other important workers who have contributed towards the study of child development. In particular Jean Piaget, in Switzerland, was originally a zoologist who later became a psychologist, and whose particular interest is cognitive behaviour and how children react and 'adapt' to their environment and experiences.

The parameters of development which Gesell described were: language, adaptive, personal-social and motor development. As a tribute to Gesell, each of these parameters, together with the measurement of hearing and vision, will be the subject of a volume in this series.

The series is written by authors who are all experts in their field but the prime aim of the series is to be practical in detail so that exponents and enthusiastic newcomers alike may be helped to practise the art. One of the fascinations of developmental paediatrics is that it combines both science and art. Science is needed in the acute accurate observation of detail and in the knowledge of the underlying principles, but art is also needed because there must be interaction between the child and the clinician in order to achieve the best motivation and performance.

It is fitting that the first volume should describe the measurement of language development. This parameter of development has long been recognized as *one* of the most important, if not *the* most important in terms of later achievement. It is generally accepted that the early detection of language handicap is most important not only for the accurate diagnosis, the differential diagnosis but, as Dr Reynell herself has shown, for therapy.

There is no doubt that perhaps the greatest contribution which preschool education can make is by stimulating verbal and communication skills. This can only be achieved following the accurate diagnosis of any delay or disorder present. This book will go a long way towards helping the clinician to make this diagnosis.

Language Development and Assessment will be of interest to a wide readership, in particular to developmental paediatricians, and to community doctors working in child health. Speech therapists, psychologists, occupational therapists and all engaged in nursery education, playgroups etc. will also find it invaluable.

Margaret Pollak
Consultant Paediatrician to the Sir Wilfrid Sheldon Assessment Centre
Senior Lecturer in Developmental, Social and Educational Paediatrics
King's College Hospital
London S.E.5

Chapter 1

INTRODUCTION AND DEFINITION OF LANGUAGE

It is intended that this book has a very practical orientation. It is based on practical experience in working with young children at a centre for handicapped children. Children with all types of handicap, including ones of specific language attended the centre, where there were classes and special programmes designed to help children who presented with early language handicaps. The stages in normal development described here are based on work concerned with the standardization of developmental language scales, which involved the assessment of large numbers of non-handicapped children from all walks of life.

The aim in writing this book is to help clinicians, who are not necessarily language specialists, to understand what is 'normal' and what is deviant in the language development of children presenting at clinics; to assess which children are in need of help; at what stage this is appropriate; and to have an understanding of the sort of help to advise.

There is now a vast amount of literature dealing with the more theoretical aspects of language development, encompassing the expertise of linguists, speech therapists, psychologists, neurologists and paediatricians. No attempt will be made here to review this literature, but there are some suggestions for further reading in Appendix III (page 169).

COMMUNICATION AND LANGUAGE

Some sort of communication between creatures of the same species is essential for corporate living. This is recognized to exist throughout the animal kingdom. Examples include the 'dance' of bees; mating rituals of birds and fish; the cries of pack animals; and the mutual 'grooming' of apes. These communications are well described by ethologists, who have studied communication patterns in detail, and show how each is built into a specific communication system, specific not only to the species, but to the situation. For example, there is a specific mating pattern of communication in birds of a particular species which requires a specific response from the partner. There is a specific communication pattern denoting territorial boundaries, which is recognized by creatures of the same species. Many of these patterns of communication are built up by using a multiplicity of clues including sound, vision, movement patterns and scent. This is a 'total' communication pattern which is also used by humans, and upon which children at the pre-language stages depend.

A mother sitting on her heels on the floor, holding out her arms, smiling, and saying 'come to Mummy', is using a pattern of communication when calling her baby to her, built up of many facets. The child responds to this pattern long before the words themselves have any meaning. The mother is using a type of communication which she adapts naturally to the level of her child's understanding. To the toddler she may call from the kitchen 'tea's ready', reducing some of the clues (such as vision and movement) but still using a phrase which is readily recognized as related to a specific situation. To school-age children she may say 'put your toys away now, its nearly teatime'; and to her husband, perhaps, 'what time will you be ready for tea?'.

In each of these examples the total communication pattern is becoming further reduced in terms of the multiplicity of clues, and increasingly dependent on the words themselves. The example 'tea's ready' has additional clues in that it is called from the kitchen, probably at the same time each day, perhaps accompanied by the smell of food, so it may be recognized as a 'situational' phrase even before words are understood. 'Put your toys away now, its nearly teatime' is beginning to use language further removed from the actual situation in that it indicates something that will happen in the immediate future. The last example, 'what time will you be ready for tea?', is making use of language for preplanning, one of the highest levels of language use, which as far as we know is only achieved by humans.

At what point does communication become true language? And how does this develop? In order to understand this, it is necessary first to define what is meant by 'language'.

DEFINITION OF LANGUAGE

A baby cries from hunger or discomfort; a dog barks at a stranger; an autistic child takes an adult's hand and puts it on something he wants. These are all forms of communication, though not actually language.

A child asks for a 'ball'; a deaf child picks up a ball in response to the appropriate hand sign for 'ball'; a child looks with understanding at a sequence of pictures in a book; older children argue about a common interest. In all these examples language is used.

In the first set of examples the communications are all 'direct', dependent on the here-and-now situation, with immediate perceptual clues. In the second set of examples they are all dependent on the use of symbols. This use of symbols is basic to true language, whatever the language form. A 'symbol' is something which can stand for or represent something else, such as a picture of a ball which may represent the object ball, or a toy table which may represent the object or concept of a table. In the examples above, the baby's cry does not stand for or represent the state of hunger, but it is a signal that the child needs immediate attention. The child asking for 'ball' is using a symbol (word) which stands for, or represents the object ball. The deaf child, following the hand sign, is understanding a different symbol which also represents the object ball, and these symbols can convey meaning even in the absence of the object they represent. The child looking at the picture book is deriving meaning from the pictures by recognizing the picture symbols as representing real objects or situations. The older children arguing are using a sophisticated form of language in which patterns of words (symbols) are used to represent ideas.

As far as we know, this ability for a highly developed symbolic understanding, flexible enough to include many forms of symbols, is specific to the human species. It is the ability to use these patterns of symbols for communication and for thinking that develops true language ability. Attempts to teach apes to use even the simplest symbols have proved laborious and slow, with only minimal achievements. Contrast this with the very rapid development of language which occurs in humans between the ages of $1\frac{1}{2}$ and 4 years. During this short time the child achieves nearly all the basic forms of verbal language, in which words become symbols for objects, and patterns of words may be formulated to represent ideas.

We can now formulate a definition of language as 'a system of symbols'. The symbols may be pictorial, hand signs, written or spoken words, or other abstract forms. They carry meaning whether or not the object that the symbol represents is present. Any of these symbolic forms may be patterned and used as language in communication with others, or used as a vehicle for thought, enabling man to transcend the here-and-now in his thinking.

Direct, non-symbolic communications are dependent on the specific situation, and the here-and-now presence of the topic of communication. Whereas the object that the autistic child wanted must be actually present and used in the communication for the meaning to be transmitted, the child asking for the 'ball' may convey the meaning whether or not the object is there.

The importance of achieving true language development will now become clear as an aspect of intellectual development as well as the more obvious importance for communication. It enables thinking and communication to go beyond the immediate situation, to plan ahead, to formulate ideas, and to work out problems.

Meaningful verbal language cannot develop until a child has reached the developmental stage of symbolic understanding which will enable him to recognize a word as standing for or representing an object or situation. How this understanding develops is described in Chapter 2.

In practical terms, when children present at clinics with problems of delayed language development, there is a need to find out first of all what stage each child has reached in the development of symbolic understanding. Is he in fact language ready? If he is not yet ready to understand verbal symbols, either for general intellectual reasons or for some more specific reason, he needs help at the appropriate prelanguage stage. In Chapter 2 the development of symbolic understanding as 'prelanguage' is described, to enable clinicians to recognize the stage at which help is needed for individual children.

Chapter 2

PRELANGUAGE

Language, defined as a system of symbols, evolves in gradual stages from situational recognition, when all the perceptual clues are present, to a truly arbitrary representational system, as verbal language, when the symbols have no perceptual similarity to their referent. In normal development this stage of the establishment of *symbolic understanding* occurs during the space of approximately 18 months, between 9 and 27 months of age. There are, of course, many further stages in the development of verbal language after this, before a mature form of language is established; these will be discussed in later chapters.

In prelanguage, so much development normally occurs during this 18-month period, each stage merging smoothly into the next, sometimes so rapidly and with so much overlap that it is not always recognized as a sequence of stages. It is only when we come into contact with handicapped children, and see how the process is often long-drawnout, that we can see more clearly the stages through which the children go.

CONCEPTS

In order to understand how 'situational understanding' develops into symbolic understanding, and so into true language, it is necessary to say something about early concept formation.

There can be no meaningful symbol until there is something in the child's understanding for the symbol to represent. He must have reached at least the early stages of concept formation before any meaningful language is possible. A concept is an inner awareness of an object, or an idea, which can be carried over when the object or situation is not present. The earliest stages of concept formation begin with the awareness of permanence of objects, the understanding that an object can continue to exist when it is no longer perceived at that moment. This can usually be demonstrated around the age of 9 months, by getting a child to search for a desired object which is momentarily hidden from him. Once a child has achieved this stage of concept formation, when he has an internalized awareness of an object even though it may not be present, he has laid the foundations for the development of symbolic understanding. He can now begin to learn that a specific symbol, as well as the actual object, can be related to the same 'concept', or internalized awareness. He learns that a picture of a chair has meaning in terms of his concept or internalized idea of a chair; or a small toy chair may also represent the idea, and so be related to the actual object.

Object perceived	$\rightarrow$	idea of object internalized as a concept; can be carried over in absence of object	$\rightarrow$	symbol of object (such as picture) related to concept and so understood to represent real object

It can be seen how much more extensive thinking and communication may become once the understanding of symbols is established.

DEVELOPMENT OF OBJECT RECOGNITION

Understanding meaningful objects begins with 'situational understanding', in the same way that early language begins. In discussing these stages of prelanguage, the development of object recognition plays an essential part. An object used in daily situations, such as a cup or spoon, will at first only be recognized within the familiar context; later these objects will have meaning apart from the specific situation in which they are used. Later still, the child will be able to generalize his concept of spoon or cup to include different types of spoon and cup, not necessarily the ones he uses daily. This is the stage of 'object recognition', when he recognizes the object as having meaning apart from the specific situation in which he encounters it daily. This object recognition, developing out of a gradual reduction of situational clues, is an essential basis for the development of symbolic understanding, and will be discussed with the prelanguage stages in this connection.

Clearly, if a child is still at the stage of recognizing only his own spoon or cup at the right time and in the right place, he is not intellectually ready to relate the word 'spoon' or 'cup' to *any* spoon or cup in *any* situation. Language can, therefore, be seen as an intellectual process, closely bound up with the stages of intellectual development, so must be discussed in this context.

SITUATIONAL UNDERSTANDING

Several months before the development of symbolic understanding children may demonstrate an understanding of familiar phrases which have been learnt as part of a regularly occurring sequence of events. Such phrases usually have a clear intonation pattern, and are used by a familiar person in a familiar situation. The child's response forms part of a well-learnt sequence of events, and demonstrates understanding which is limited to this context. A common example is 'clap hands', or 'do pat-a-cake', when a child is suitably positioned on his mother's knee, and she may even clap her own hands first. At this stage of understanding the child responds appropriately to the right person in the right situation, if the phrase is said according to the learnt tonal pattern, but the individual words themselves have no meaning. The phrase is only meaningful as part of a familiar sequence of events, and is in no way representational or symbolic.

The same thing happens in terms of vocalization, with expressive jargon. A child uses intonation patterns and rhythms which simulate phrases in certain daily situations. A child of 18 months, for example, was heard using jargon simulating his mother's cross voice when she was annoyed with him for not settling down to bed at night. There are no recognizable words, but the phrase pattern may be situationally appropriate.

DEVELOPMENT FROM SITUATIONAL UNDERSTANDING THROUGH TO SYMBOLIC UNDERSTANDING

Figure 1 shows how preverbal language is related to and paced by a more generalized symbolic understanding.

At the stage of situational understanding, it is the total situation, with all the familiar perceptual clues, that communicates the meaning to the child. The phrase or object forms part of a familiar perceptual sequence which the child first learns to recognize with evidence of anticipation, and then to respond to with appropriate action so that his own response becomes part of the familiar sequence. In the case of object recognition, it may be certain aspects such as the handle or topological shape of the cup that have special significance within the perceptual sequence. This merges into true object recognition when the

Prelanguage

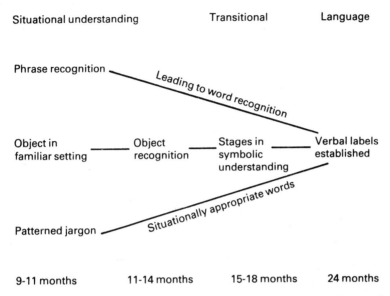

Figure 1   How preverbal language is related to and paced
by a more generalized symbolic understanding

cup is recognized without situational clues. In the same
way, the word 'cup' may become the significant word in a
phrase regularly associated with the situation of drinking
from a cup; this word may later elicit the whole drinking
sequence, and finally be related specifically to the object
cup.

These stages are set out in more detail in Table 1, which
shows how a familiar situation develops into object recognition, and then progresses through the early stages of
symbolic understanding, to evolve as a verbal label, which
is true language.

What is actually happening is a gradual reduction first
in the total situational clues, and then in the non-linguistic
perceptual clues. In other words, the symbol becomes less
perceptually similar to the object or situation it stands for,
so must begin to be recognized without these aids. Percep-

Table 1 The development of symbolic understanding

Stage	Approximate age level	Stage description	Example	Behaviour manifestation
1	8–9 months	Confined situational recognition	Own cup recognized in usual situation at usual time	Excited anticipation
2	9–10 months	Extended situational recognition	Own cup recognized in different setting but still with some familiar clues such as having bib on	Anticipation with attempts to drink
3	10–11 months	Situational recognition with some generalization	Own cup recognized in any situation	Drinking activities
4	11–12 months	Pre-object recognition	Recognizes other cups of same size but with small perceptual differences, in a few different settings	Drinking activities, possibly after some hesitation
5	12–13 months	True object recognition	Understanding of object extended to any 'real'-sized cup in any setting	'Drinks' from cup without hesitation even if cup is empty

	Age			
6	13–15 months	Early symbolic recognition	Understanding of Wendy House-sized cup as representing object cup	Drinking or 'pretend' drinking
7	15–17 months	Relating two easy symbols	Understands relationship of toy cup to doll or teddy bear	Pretends feeding doll or teddy bear from cup
8	18–20 months	Recognition of more remote three-dimensional symbols	Recognizes representation when more perceptual clues are withdrawn, such as small doll play	Feeding actions with dolls' house toys
9	20–24 months	Recognition of two-dimensional symbols	Recognition of clear coloured pictures	Relates object to picture
10	24–27 months	Relates two different types of symbol	Matches small toys to pictures	After demonstration, can match toys and pictures representing familiar objects
11	2½+ years	Using concrete symbols as 'language' to express connected ideas	Acting out simple sequences with small toys	Imaginative play with small toys, creating story sequences
12	4+ years	Using two-dimensional symbols as language	Constructing meaningful picture sequences	Puts together picture stores, understands comic strips

tual clues such as size and shape are most easily recognized visually, but they also have a tactile component. The same sequence could be traced in terms of other auditory and tactile clues, but this is often less easy and less direct.

The stages set out in Table 1 show how the total situational clues are gradually reduced to the stage at which object recognition occurs (stage 5). At this stage the child has a true internalized object concept of a cup, so that any object which fits this category is recognized as appropriate for drinking. Once object recognition is established, the ground is prepared for the development of symbols.

This development of symbols implies a further generalization to include not only other objects of the same type, but also representations of the object. The perceptual clues are gradually reduced in this process of moving from recognition of real objects to an understanding of an arbitrary symbol such as a verbal label. In assessment and teaching it is usually best to vary attributes such as size and colour first, keeping to three-dimensional material, for example moving from a real object, perhaps a white china cup, to a Wendy House-sized plastic toy cup which may be pink or blue. When recognition of doll's house-sized toys is established, children are ready for two-dimensional work, so moving on to pictures.

A verbal label usually has little perceptual similarity to the object it represents, so it is not until fairly late in the whole sequence that an understanding of verbal labels can be established. Table 2 shows the sequence.

Verbal language can be considered to have begun when a word is definitely related to an object as a true label, in other words, when it has become a medium of symbols. The stages leading up to this are all prelanguage. It is important to recognize this distinction. If attempts are made to get children to 'talk' and to name objects before they are symbolically ready, the words will be used or

Prelanguage

Table 2 How the stages in the development of symbolic understanding relate to the stages in preverbal language development

Stage	Preverbal language
1	Early situational understanding, phrase recognition
2 to 3	Extension of phrase recognition with some appropriate responses Expressive jargon simulating phrases
4 to 5	Identification of words within phrases in familiar settings, such as 'time for a drink, here's your *cup*', expressive jargon patterns become situationally linked, with some attempt to imitate specific words
6 to 8	Beginning to understand object labels, selects a few objects in response to naming Uses a few words, mainly situational words such as 'no', 'ta', and 'bye-bye'
8 to 9	Achievement of true verbal labels; prelanguage merges into 'language'
10 to 12	Increasing elaboration of receptive and expressive verbal language

recognized only when the other clues are present. An apparent understanding of the word 'cup' may occur when this is asked for always in the same situation, but it may not be used or understood without the familiar situational back-up. This situation-bound talk occurs particularly in some mentally handicapped children or autistic children, who may have a superficial speech fluency; it can interfere with true language learning. Children who are not ready for true language need to be taught at the prelanguage stages, starting at whatever stage the child has reached.

Very early help, therefore, is advised for all children whose language development is delayed, at whatever stage, including the prelanguage stages described here.

Chapter 3

NORMAL DEVELOPMENT OF VERBAL LANGUAGE

Discussion in the previous chapter traced how, in normal development, true language evolves from total communication patterns and situational understanding. The situational clues are gradually dispensed with until the symbols alone have specific meaning. These symbols can then be combined into sequences, so forming meaningful patterns of 'language' communication which transcends the here-and-now situation and is no longer dependent on the actual presence of the object referents.

We can now trace the early stages in the development of verbal language. This is the most highly developed form of symbolic communication, when the symbols (words) bear little or no perceptual similarity to their referents.

The sequence of stages in the development of verbal comprehension and expressive language is fairly consistent, as it is determined by the stages in intellectual development upon which it depends. It is the intellectual basis which also determines the rate at which true verbal language develops in normal children. We have seen, in Chapter 2, how concept formation must precede symbolic understanding, and how symbolic understanding is an essential prerequisite of true verbal language. Some understanding and use of familiar phrase patterns may develop earlier, but these are situation-bound and are not part of true language as defined here. The sequence of developmental stages is usually the same for verbal comprehension and expressive language, but expressive language develops a little later, so both aspects will be discussed together when describing the developmental stages. The age levels at which some of the stages are usually achieved are indicated in Table 3 on page 32. The overall pattern of development, relating both aspects of verbal language to the more central aspects of intellectual understanding, including symbolic understanding, is illustrated in Figure 2.

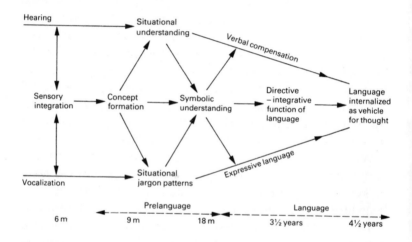

Figure 2   The integration of some processes involved in the development of verbal language

EARLY PHRASE PATTERNS

When asked what were the first words used or understood by a child, the answer is often 'ee-ar' (here you are); 'all-gone'; 'bye-bye'; or 'more'. Is this true language in the sense of symbolic representation? These early phrases, either understood as 'verbal comprehension' or used as 'expressive language', are usually linked to specific situations, and form part of a well-learnt sequence of events. 'Ee-ar' is usually first understood as relating to the sequence of transferring an object from one person to another, and apart from this situational context it has no meaning. It accompanies, but does not represent, this act of transference. The same could apply to the other examples given. 'By-bye' is associated with the situation of leave-taking and somebody waving a hand. Children learn to respond to this total communication pattern by waving their own hand. It is not easy to draw a clear line between this sort of prelanguage and true words as symbolic representations, but when a verbal label is understood as belonging to a specific meaningful object, wherever that object is, then verbal language has begun. Using the definition given on page 16, of language as a system of symbols, true verbal language begins with the first verbal label. If a child can select a spoon from a choice of three or more objects, in response to the word 'spoon', in situations where the spoon is not necessarily used, then he has established a connection between the word and the object; the *word* 'spoon' is clearly established as a symbol representing the *object* spoon.

There is a precarious stage before this, when the word is not yet firmly attached to the object, and still depends on a few situational clues. A mother often expresses surprise and disappointment when her child fails to select the spoon in a test situation. She may say, 'I can't understand it, he knows it at home'. So he probably does, but the unfamiliar setting is enough to loosen the precarious attachment of word and object so that he cannot do this in a test situation. He may select it correctly occasionally but not consistently. This gives the examiner some indication of the level of consolidation he has reached in this stage of understanding.

Table 3 Approximate ages at which some of the stages described in the text are acquired

Approximate age	Symbolic understanding (non-verbal language)	Verbal comprehension	Expressive verbal language
8–10 months	Early concept formation Awareness of permanence of objects	Some situational understanding of phrase patterns	Patterned vocalization
12 months	Object recognition	Appropriate response to familiar phrases	Expressive jargon
15–18 months	Early symbolic recognition Large doll-play	A few verbal labels understood	Uses a few recognizable words
18–21 months	Basic symbolic understanding established Small doll-play Recognises clear coloured pictures	Selects familiar objects in response to naming	Vocabulary of 12+ words
2–2½ years	Relates symbol to symbol Matches toys to pictures	Relates two named objects 'put the *spoon* in the *cup*'	Names familiar objects Word combinations
2½–3 years	Understands more arbitrary symbols Relates gesture to picture	Selects objects by use 'which do we cook with?'	Uses short sentences including prepositions and pronouns
3–4 years		Follows increasingly complex verbal directions containing three to four 'operative' words per sentence	Fluent sentences – usually of mature structure by 4 years

THE FIRST OBJECT LABELS

The first words learnt may vary with different early experiences and in different cultures, so any generalizations made here must be understood to refer to the standardization sample for the Reynell Developmental Language Scales (Reynell, 1977 ref). English children were used in this sample, mainly from South-East England including the London area, but with a small sample from the North of the country.

The earliest labels are concerned with familiar objects in everyday use, especially those which have particular significance for the child, such as a favourite toy (for instance, a teddy) or objects associated with mealtimes. 'Spoon', 'ball' and 'car' are among the earliest words understood as verbal labels. At this early stage the word 'car' is usually referred to a toy car rather than to the real object. There may, in fact, be no connection in the child's understanding between the two. The word 'cup' is usually understood a little later because it is often referred to as 'drinkie' or 'mug'. In teaching early language it is advisable to use the same word always for the same object, as two different words can confuse the child at the early stages of verbal labels.

At this early stage a child can only assimilate one 'operative' word or concept at a time. His understanding may include whole phrases, such as 'put it down', or a single verbal label as in 'where's the ball?'. When talking to children it is more natural to put the operative word into a short sentence such as 'where's the ball?' or 'here's your ball', but the understanding will only be related to the single concept 'ball'.

WORD COMBINATIONS

It is not until a little later, at 2–2$\frac{1}{4}$ years, that children learn to assimilate and relate two operative words at a time, such as 'put the *ball* in the *box*'', or 'all-gone ball'. Linguistically these examples are different types of construction, but from the intellectual point of view they still represent examples of assimilating two concepts, whether these are object concepts (verbal labels) or situational concepts such as 'all-gone'. It is no accident, developmentally, that this is also the age at which a child can relate two different types of symbol to the same concept, in matching a toy to a picture. This two-concept stage is also evident in expressive language at about the same age in the use of word combinations. The child deliberately brings together two meaningful words, or a word and phrase, such as 'bye-bye Daddy'; 'Daddy gone'.

In all these three aspects of language there is a bringing together and relating of two separate symbols, relating them in a meaningful way. In verbal comprehension a child assimilated two operative words in following the direction 'put the ball in the box'. He does not, at this early stage, understand the back-up words such as 'in', and would still put the ball in the box even if the direction was 'put the ball under the box'. In matching a toy to a picture (such as toy chair to picture of chair) he is relating two different types of symbol representing the same concept. This is a non-verbal relationship of symbols which demonstrates a verbal language readiness at the two-concept stage (2–2¼ years). In using word combinations by bringing together two separate words or phrases in expressive language, he is again making a meaningful relationship between two symbols.

This is the second important developmental stage, when the stage of single verbal labels moves on to simple meaningful combinations of two separate symbols or words.

NOUN–VERB STAGE

By the age of about 2½ years children are able to extend their understanding of language to include a noun–verb combination which goes further than situational understanding. The understanding of verbs is more difficult than the understanding of nouns, as they are perceptually less clearly defined. A ball is a ball, and is labelled 'ball'. The object 'ball' can be perceived clearly and has very consistent characteristics. But what of 'running', 'sleeping', 'sitting'? These are action words with less clearly defined dimensions, and which cannot have meaning in the absence of a subject to demonstrate the actions. Intellectually this involves a higher level of conceptualization, and so is a later stage in language development than is the understanding of verbal labels, either singly or combined. The fact that a verb can have no meaning apart from its link with a subject, either stated or implied, means that children must at least have reached the stage of two-concept understanding (described on page 34) in order to reach the stage of understanding verbs as actions. Verbs as 'situational' understanding may occur earlier, as in 'Daddy gone', or 'ee-ar ball'; but a verb used as a clearly defined and specific action is more difficult.

If we relate the stages of language development all the time to the intellectual implications, the developmental progress can be well understood, and a rational teaching programme planned.

The earliest verbs understood relate to actions that the child can do himself, and so has immediate first-hand experience of them. These include activities such as 'sit', 'run', 'sleep', 'drink', and 'play'. As with the first verbal labels, it is the early personal experience which determines the order in which the actual words are learnt, but once the particular stage of understanding is reached, the vocabulary at that stage increases rapidly.

STAGE OF THREE OR MORE CONCEPTS AND SIMPLE SENTENCES

Between 2½ and 4 years of age there is a very rapid advance in language development. During this time children become able to follow directions which include three or more 'operative' words, such as 'fetch Daddy's shoes', 'put the spoon and the fork on the plate', 'put the button under the cup', 'find the big red brick'. From these examples it can be seen that, at this three-concept stage, the words begin to extend beyond nouns and verbs, and include more advanced understanding using prepositions and adjectives.

The understanding of the words must again wait for the understanding of the concept. It is of no use to teach a child the word 'big' until he has an understanding of the concepts of 'big' and 'small', or 'big' and 'little'. These words are often expected too early, so that they become associated with a specific person or object rather than understood as a symbol for the abstractions relating to relative size. Children may learn 'little boy' or 'big daddy' before they understand what big and little really mean in terms of a concept which can be transferred to other things. It is not until 2¾ years of age that children can sort objects into two simple categories such as big and small, so demonstrating an understanding of the concept as such. Until they can do this type of sorting, the word is not going to be understood in its true meaning as a symbol for the attribute of size or colour, or whatever concept is referred to. In teaching deviant children it is important to link the language with the actual conceptual understanding, as they may be very out of step one way or another. Words such as 'big' and 'small' should be taught alongside simple sorting tasks so that the concept is learnt and labelled at the same time. In normal development children come through to an understanding of the concepts through daily living and play experiences, but it is always as well to be aware of the need for understanding the concept before expecting an understanding or use of the words.

The same thing applies to any words describing abstract concepts, whether these are describing position (in/out; up/down; beside/behind); colour, shape, or any other of the apparently simple words we often expect children to understand much too soon. These words are often understood only when linked to specific situations or specific objects such as 'red ball', or 'in bed', giving a false impression of the child's true understanding of the concept.

Pronouns come relatively late. It is quite difficult for a child to sort out 'I', 'me', 'you', 'his' etc. Parents understand this and usually adapt their own speech naturally, by saying things such as 'that's Bobby's ball', 'this is Mummy's hat'. This is quite appropriate for children under 2½ years. After that there is a transitional stage when the following examples may be appropriate for teaching: 'It's your ball. . . . Bobby's ball', 'it's my hat. . . . Mummy's hat'. This helps the child to understand the pronouns by giving the immediate referent. It is not until 3 years that most children can use pronouns consistently and appropriately, although 'me' and 'mine' may be used earlier.

It is not possible to give exact age levels, or even a reliable order of development for the understanding and use of words representing these more abstract concepts, as this will vary according to the different experiences of children and with their rate and pattern of intellectual development. The important thing is to understand the close relationship between the development of language and the intellectual understanding upon which it depends.

USE OF PAST AND FUTURE TENSES

Understanding and use of past tenses comes before that of future tenses. Again, this follows the intellectual pattern. The immediate past is part of the child's actual experience, and so more readily becomes part of his understanding than something which has not yet happened. Both involve the ability to use language to transcend the here and now, and so already represent a relatively advanced language ability.

Parents are often surprised that 5 year old children cannot tell them what they had for lunch at school, or what they did in school that morning. It is often assumed that they are unwilling to tell, but in fact the children are being asked to use language in a way that is quite beyond them. To recapitulate a past experience, and translate it into descriptive language, however simple the language, is a hard task for a 5 year old. It is better, in the early stages, to ask about an immediate happening when there are still some perceptual clues. For example, in play with toy cars, one may crash into another, and the child could be asked 'what happened?'. The actual presence of the cars can help him to reconstruct the past action and put it into words.

A consistent and appropriate use of future tenses is not expected until 4 to 4½ years of age. This involves one of the highest levels of language use in thinking ahead and preplanning. There is nothing concrete to 'hold on to' in talking about things that have not yet happened, so the language must stand on its own. In our thinking this becomes one of the greatest intellectual assets – the ability to use an internalized symbolic form for thinking out problems and ideas, planning 'what will happen if . . .'. This sort of thinking is, of course, possible without verbal language, but internalized verbal language vastly increases the scope of thought. This intellectual aspect of language is one of the main reasons for concern about children who are seriously delayed in language development. There is a danger that, if things are not put right at an early stage, there could be limitations later on in the aspects of intellectual development that depend on language.

INTELLECTUAL USE OF LANGUAGE

We now come to perhaps the most important aspect of language development which is the process of integrating language with other aspects of intellectual development so that the whole may be increasingly productive.

In the early stages of verbal understanding children have difficulty in integrating verbal directions with a practical activity. If a child under 2 years is attempting a practical task such as building a tower of bricks, an adult giving directions such as 'put another one on top', is likely to be more of a distraction than a help. The child's attention is on the practical aspects of the task and his verbal understanding is too uncertain for directions to be helpful. He must either ignore them or leave what he is doing and attempt to listen. When playing with children at this developmental stage it is best for very simple comments to accompany the activity rather than precede it – for example: 'This brick goes on top, see', while matching the action to the phrase.

Between the ages of $2\frac{1}{2}$ and $3\frac{1}{2}$ years children can be helped by simple verbal directions immediately preceding the activity, such as 'Here's another brick, put it on top'. Children are now beginning to integrate verbal directions with a practical activity which is ongoing, in such a way that the directions help them to work out the practical task. This can be seen, too, when children are attempting simple form boards. If the examiner says 'turn it round', or 'try another hole', this may help the child to succeed in the task. In most test procedures this sort of direction will invalidate the standard score, but it does give the examiner useful information about the stage of development in linking language with practical activities.

By about 3½ years of age children begin to direct their own activities verbally, by talking aloud about what they are doing or immediately intending to do. They may be heard to do this while carrying out a form board task if they name the pieces, 'like a ball' . . . 'like a window', or if they direct themselves 'no, not that . . . goes here'. In doing simple block designs they may direct themselves with guidance such as 'nuther one here . . . blue one now'. They are now definitely using language in thinking and this is helping them to work out practical problems in the here-and-now situation. At first this self-direction must be said aloud, but by about 4½ to 5 years of age it becomes internalized so that the child only has to 'think' the verbal directions in order for this to be of help in whatever activity he is engaged upon. There is usually a transitional whispering stage, which may even be sub-auditory. When verbal guidance is internalized, language has become a truly intellectual medium, forming the important language–performance link which becomes the basis for so much subsequent intellectual development.

This development can be seen working through the stages, in observing children's play. Quite young children, in the early stages of learning object labels, will attempt to stabilize their own object concepts by naming the objects as they handle them. They may also accompany their play with appropriate noises (car noises, for instance), and later by an abbreviated commentary, which adds an extra dimension to the play and consolidates the ideas they are working out. Language is beginning to integrate different aspects of their activities. Later still, at about 3½ years of age, language immediately precedes the action, so that it is now becoming part of the planning and directing aspect of thinking. This leads to more silent play as the directive function of language is finally internalized as verbal thinking. As maturation proceeds, the interval of time between planning and action may be lengthened, and eventually the concrete material may be dispensed with, so that internalized planning may take over the role of trial and error with concrete material. This final stage does not occur until well into school age.

Delays and deviations in language development may occur at any of the developmental stages, from the earliest stages of situational prelanguage and symbolic under-standing, to the higher levels of complex sentences. Some indications of the sort of problems that may occur with children referred to developmental clinics are discussed in the following chapters.

Chapter 4

DEVELOPMENTAL LANGUAGE DELAYS AND DEVIATIONS

This is not intended to be a book about the different types of language handicap, but rather a guide to clinicians on how to assess what is normal and what needs help; so this chapter will be concerned only in a general way with the range of language handicaps likely to be encountered in developmental clinics. The problems will be related to the stages in development described in previous chapters, as this will aid the clinician in understanding the developmental stages at which help is appropriate for a particular child.

Figure 2 on page 30 illustrates the developmental aspect.

Table 4   Grouping of language handicaps

(a) *Central intellectual*	(b) *Verbal language, central*	(c) *Verbal language, peripheral*
Mental retardation	Developmental language delay	Environmental
Problems in symbolic understanding, autistic type	Developmental language deviations	Articulation Muscular control
Problems of attention and listening		Hearing

A useful scheme for clinicians in development clinics is illustrated in Table 4. The presenting language handicap may be part of a more extensive problem, as in the conditions included under the first heading, 'central intellectual'. Here the contributory cause, or perhaps the main cause, is not directly due to a verbal language difficulty, but rather the verbal language difficulty is due to some more basic cause which itself needs help. These children have problems very early in the developmental sequence (illustrated in Figure 2).

More specific handicaps may be related to verbal language development under the second heading 'Verbal language, central'. These, too, are intellectual problems, as language itself is part of a child's intellectual make up, as explained above in Chapter 3. The handicap in these children affects a later stage of development, with the more basic aspects of intellect and symbolic understanding relatively unaffected. The difficulty may involve both verbal comprehension and expressive language; or perhaps only one of these aspects may be primarily involved.

Under the third heading, the language problem is secondary to more peripheral handicaps, with the more central aspects of language being potentially normal.

It should be understood that these headings are only intended as a guide to assessment. To some extent the separation, particularly of the first two headings, is artificial, as there is great overlap and interaction between all developing intellectual and linguistic processes. There is often involvement of some of the aspects included under the first heading, even when the main problem is a specifically verbal one. In our own sample of preschool children, presenting with early language handicaps, 50 per cent also had problems of attention, and 27 per cent had problems involving symbolic understanding and/or concept formation. It is, therefore, important that any young child presenting with early language handicaps should have a very thorough assessment including all aspects of early intellectual development.

PROBLEMS OF ATTENTION AND LISTENING

The development of attention control is closely bound up with language development, as it is with any learning. It is particularly relevant to language development because language learning requires a more mature level of attention control than does learning from concrete material. Many children presenting with early language delay have been found to have immature attention control, and remedial work on attention problems has helped the children to develop language (Cooper *et al.*, 1974).

Experience of working with handicapped children has indicated certain definite stages in the development of attention control, which can be recognized during the assessment. A study of non-handicapped children (Reynell, 1977) has confirmed that these are true developmental stages and has indicated approximate age levels for each stage. There is considerable variability, as attention depends to some extent on the situation, and on the nature of the task attempted, but the progression of the stages in development seems clear, and can be a useful teaching guide. The following six developmental stages occur between the ages of 0 to 6 years.

First stage

First is the stage of extreme distractability which is normal in the first year of life. The child's attention is held momentarily by whatever is the dominant stimulus in the environment, and he is easily distracted by any new stimulus. Examples of such intrusive stimuli which may occur during the assessment are someone walking by in the corridor; a car hooter outside; the examiner picking up a pencil or turning over a paper. In teaching children who are at this stage, control of the learning environment is of the greatest importance. The learning task must be the dominant stimulus, with other distractions reduced to a minimum. Behaviour at this stage of fleeting attention may range from extreme hyperactivity, to those lethargic children whose interest drifts away every few seconds. Also included in this group are those atypical and often very disturbed children who are distracted by their own fantasies, so that attention to learning tasks is fleeting.

Second stage

At this stage, normally occurring in the second year of life, a child can concentrate for some time on a concrete task of his own choice. This is rigid and inflexible, particularly at first, probably because attention is so precariously held that all other stimuli must be cut out in order to sustain it. Such children cannot use, or even tolerate any intervention or attempts to modify the task by an adult, whether this is verbal or visual. This is a threatened interfering stimulus which must be cut out. At this stage children are sometimes described as 'obstinate', if the reasons for their rigid, self-directed and non-cooperative behaviour is not understood. They are not easy to teach, because the directions cannot be related to the task unless they form an intrinsic part of the learning task itself. Children at this stage usually enjoy tasks such as form boards and picture puzzles, where the directions are implicit in the task, and success is self-evident. Rewards too, must be part of the task, and not something which happens afterwards. At this stage a child cannot appreciate that he will get a sweet as a result of a particular action (unless this has been specifically taught). If his attention is on the sweet, this is what he must have here and now. If learning tasks can be so arranged that the reward is part of the task itself, then the reward is effective – for example, putting a sweet inside a nest of boxes in order to get the child to carry out a manipulative task with the boxes.

Third stage

At this stage, usually in the third year of life, attention is becoming a little more flexible, but it is still 'single-channelled'. In other words the child's whole attention, visual and auditory, must be on the source of the directions. He cannot assimilate verbal directions, for example, if he is fiddling with toys. He must stop what he is doing and look at the speaker. The attention focus is more flexible in that, with adult help, he can now shift the focus from task to directions and then back to the task. At this stage the control of the attention focus is entirely with the adult, as the child cannot yet control this for himself. Before any directions are given, whether these are verbal or by demonstration, his attention focus must be set so that he is giving his full attention, auditory and visual, to the directions being given. He then needs help in transferring the directions immediately to the task. In teaching such children it is important to make sure the child is sitting still, without fiddling with toys or other teaching material, and that he is looking at the speaker's face. He can only assimilate the directions if his whole attention is on the source from which they come, whether this is verbal or by demonstration.

Fourth stage

During the fourth year of life most children can begin to control their own attention focus. Attention is still single-channelled, so that a child must give his full attention, visual and auditory, to any directions given to him, but he does this spontaneously and under his own control, without needing to have his attention set by an adult before each verbal direction is given. He moves gradually towards a stage where he only needs to look at the speaker when the directions become difficult for him to understand.

Fifth and sixth stages

This is the stage of school readiness where a child can assimilate verbal directions related to the task he is engaged upon, without needing to interrupt the task to look at the speaker. This two-channelled attention, integrating auditory and visual (or manipulatory) learning, is at first sustained only for short periods, after which the interest of one or other aspect takes over. When children have reached this stage of attention control they are ready for teaching in a class, where directions are often given to the class as a whole, while the children are carrying out some practical activity such as drawing or building.

The sixth stage is mature school entry level, where integrated attention is well established and well sustained.

Although a good deal of useful learning about concrete material can proceed at attention level 2, the more mature levels of stages 3 and 4 are needed for language learning. A child needs to be able to focus his full attention on the speaker and then carry over the directions to whatever he is doing. This can proceed in a one-to-one situation, under adult control, at attention level 3, and more securely at stage 4, when the child is beginning to control his own attention focus.

It is important for clinicians to understand the close connection between language development and the developmental level of attention control. It is easy to say 'he couldn't do it because he doesn't listen', but this may be a gross oversimplification of the problem, and miss the real cause of the difficulty which needs help. It is more likely that he *cannot* listen, because his attention level is not mature enough to cope with what is being asked of him. This sort of difficulty should be carefully assessed so that appropriate help may be given.

DEVELOPMENTAL LANGUAGE DELAY

This is a constitutionally determined developmental handicap. It may be mild or severe, and may or may not be associated with evidence of a more generally handicapping condition. This amounts to a handicap needing special help when receptive and/or expressive language development is not more than two-thirds of the non-verbal intellectual ability level in terms of age equivalent. Although this is a serious and pathological delay, the language, when it appears, follows a fairly consistent developmental pattern, with the normal stages of early language development. The natural history of this type of language delay is for verbal comprehension and expressive language to be approximately equally delayed at first, often with very immature attention control. Verbal comprehension recovers first, then the more central aspects of expressive language (words and sentences), and finally the more mature coding of sounds in words (intelligibility) Early intonation patterns, and the stages of development of speech sounds are usually normal, but delayed in these children.

The pattern of language handicap presenting at assessment will depend on the stage at which the child is seen. In the early stages, receptive and expressive aspects will be approximately equally retarded; but if the first referral takes place when some early resolution has already occurred, the expressive language may appear to be much more retarded than verbal comprehension, masking the fact that verbal comprehension still needs help.

Although some of these children may resolve their difficulties spontaneously in time, it is important to provide help as soon as the difficulty is recognized. Spontaneous resolution will, at best, be very delayed, so denying the child the use of language at the age he is needing it as part of his intellectual development.

DEVIANT LANGUAGE DEVELOPMENT

These children also have a severe and specific language delay, but the pattern of their language is also deviant. There is no clear pattern of recovery, as in developmental language delay, but development is uneven and atypical. The handicap may be very specifically concerned with one aspect of language, for example a specific type of receptive or expressive difficulty. The handicap is sometimes difficult to overcome completely. The children usually make good early progress, with help, but complete recovery tends to be slower than in the developmental language delays, and the children may enter school with a disability still severe enough to need ongoing help.

Children with a severe and specific verbal comprehension difficulty may present as self-absorbed non-listeners. They may have a good deal of superficial chatter, which can be misleading in terms of the severity of the handicap, until their utterances are carefully examined. These utterances may be found to consist of a number of well-learnt catch phrases, used appropriately enough, but at a 'situational' level. The sentences are slotted in to the appropriate daily situations, but are invariable in pattern. The sentences or phrases are usually a direct imitation of adult speech, learnt as a whole without assimilating the meaning. Although at first it may sound as though these children have relatively mature language, a closer examination reveals severe problems with semantics. An example was Helen, a four-year-old, mildly retarded child, who constantly played with dolls, repeating phrases such as 'dolly have a drink', 'put dolly to bed now', all said at the appropriate time in play, but never varying, and never extended. Helen could not understand or follow the simplest verbal directions unless they were already built into her daily repertoire. Such children are in urgent need of help, as it is only too easy for them to develop a fluent and relatively meaningless superficial 'speech'.

There are other types of primarily verbal comprehension difficulties, but a full discussion would be beyond the scope of this volume. Clinicians will be alerted to the existence of such difficulties, however, by regular assessment of verbal comprehension in all children presenting with language handicaps.

The range of specific expressive language handicaps is extensive, both in type and degree, but again a full discussion would be out of place here. The clinician should, however, be able to assess the seriousness of the difficulty in terms of the need for help. From the developmental point of view, difficulties may occur at any of the stages shown in Figure 2. They may be at the early stage of verbal labels, when children cannot find the words they want, perhaps even in naming simple everyday objects. They may be able to produce the correct sound association, such as 'brm-brm' for a car, 'sh-sh' for water, or a hum for the carpet sweeper, but the actual symbol (word) is hard or impossible for them to produce. Other children may persist at the jargon stage, so that their utterances, although appropriately patterned in terms of tone and rhythm, are not intelligible in terms of words. The latter is more common in developmental language delay than in language deviances. Children may fail at the later developmental stage of sentence construction, so that their ideas are expressed in 'lumps' made up of a telegraphic type of sentence or phrase. At a still later developmental stage, the children have achieved the stage of words and simple sentences, but have difficulty in coding sounds in words. These children are usually able to make the sounds in isolation, but use consonant substitutions when speaking. Although their sentences may be quite good, they are often unintelligible unless the context is known.

All these difficulties, including delayed and deviant language, may show considerable overlap, and the pattern may change as the child gets older, so the divisions do not reflect clear diagnostic categories. They are intended more as a descriptive guide. As far as providing help is concerned, one thing seems clear, and that is that children with all types and degrees of early central language problems are in urgent need of help. The more severe the handicap, the more urgent the need, particularly if the difficulty involves verbal comprehension. Work has shown (Cooper *et al.*, 1978) that appropriate early help is rewarding with all central language difficulties when the remedial programme is directed towards the basic stages of language development which are common to all cases, and if work is adjusted to the appropriate developmental stages which are revealed at assessment.

VERBAL LANGUAGE, PERIPHERAL

Environmental language delay

This is exactly what it says, that is, a language delay which is due entirely to environmental circumstances in an otherwise normal child. Deprivation of language experience must be severe in order to cause a significant language delay, and this is not often encountered now in this country. Most parents spend time with their children, at least in the daily care of feeding, bathing and dressing, and this affords opportunities for communication and language learning. There are a few cases, however, in which this early language and communication experience does not occur, or is inadequate, such as with deaf-mute parents; with some of the children put out to 'child minders'; with the rare parents who do not talk to their children; or with children left alone for long periods. There are also problems, sometimes, with immigrant children, who settle in a country where the language is not their native tongue, during the formative years of language development.

This type of language delay is not often severe, and usually recovers spontaneously with the provision of suitable early language experience. A good nursery school or day nursery with a high staff ratio can do a great deal to help these children.

Problems due to anatomical malformations

Clinicians should be alerted to the possibility of difficulty in speech production resulting from causes such as unusual dentition or abnormal palate formation. This is a specialist subject, not concerned with central (intellectual) aspects of language development, so any further discussion here would be out of place. Indications of such difficulties, from the point of view of language development, may be a difficulty in producing certain sounds, whether in words or in isolation, or difficulties with voicing and phonation. This is in contrast to the 'coding' difficulty referred to on page 52, where the sounds can be made in isolation but are wrongly coded in words, when the children use consonant substitutions. The latter is a central language difficulty and not a mechanical one.

Verbal comprehension and expressive language development should be normal in these children if there is no central language problem as well. It is well known, however, that malformations are more common in children who have extensive handicaps, perhaps including mental retardation, than in otherwise normal children, so even when the presenting difficulty seems to be a purely mechanical one, the clinician should not dismiss the possibility of some central involvement without a full assessment.

Problems in speech production due to difficulties in muscular control

This type of difficulty, sometimes referred to as 'dysarthria', is common in children who suffer from cerebral palsy or any other condition affecting the control of speech musculature. Neurological conditions of this sort usually involve extensive handicaps. In the case of cerebral palsy, and other conditions where the cause is cerebral, there is likely to be some central language problem as well as the more obvious one of difficulty in speech production, so once again, a full assessment, especially of verbal comprehension is important. There is a need to know how much understanding a child has, even if he cannot produce any recognizable words. It may be that he will need to be taught an alternative system of verbal expression.

Hearing difficulties

This is so obviously a cause of language delay that it may seem redundant to mention it here. It is worth stressing, however, that even a mild hearing impairment, or a transient one, can have a considerable effect on language development if it is present during the formative years of $1\frac{1}{2}$–4.

Chapter 5

ASSESSMENT OF THE STAGES IN PRELANGUAGE DEVELOPMENT

AIMS

Having discussed the development of language in previous chapters, and its significance in relation to other aspects of intellectual development, we now come to the more practical issues of how to assess this in individual children presenting at developmental clinics.

First of all the aims of assessment should be defined because this will determine the type of assessment carried out. The aim is, literally, to 'assess' the present position with a view to providing immediate and appropriate help. This is different from aiming to 'diagnose' or 'categorize' with a view to predicting future implications. Diagnosis is obviously important as far as the total paediatric condition is concerned, and other factors such as hearing, social and emotional problems will also need a full investigation, but from the point of view of language development this is an 'assessment' of the here and now position, with a view to immediate help. It is only the assessment of language development that comes within the scope of this volume.

The aim, as defined above, makes an assumption that it is possible to provide help for all types of language handicap. In some cases the difficulty may not be completely resolved, but at least we can aim for each child to develop such potential as he has. We aim to assess the present position in relation to all aspects of language and communication, and the present level and rate of development, as this will provide an appropriate starting-point for help, and enable a programme of help to be individually tailored to each child's needs. It is not helpful, for example, to try to teach a child to say words when he still has no understanding of more primitive symbols such as small toys and pictures. It is also unhelpful to label him as not yet language-ready, or too young for speech therapy. Appropriate help can be given at any stage, including the prelanguage stages, provided it is at the right stage for that particular child. Help is directed towards consolidating the stage the child has reached, in different aspects of language development, and helping him towards the next stage. It is all too easy to say 'we will try this' or 'try that' and see if it helps, without direct relation to the relevant developmental stages. This can result in wasting important developmental months, or even years for the child. It is vital to provide the right sort of help as soon as possible in order to make the optimum use of the developmental time available for young children. Concern to teach certain speech sounds such as 's' and 'r', is quite inappropriate, for example, in a child who can only produce about six words spontaneously. Concern to get him to imitate, 'say ball', 'say biscuit', etc., when his verbal comprehension is so limited that he cannot even select these items in response to naming, is also inappropriate, and can only lead to meaningless 'speech'.

The clinician who first assesses the child will need to have enough understanding to give some immediate advice to the parents, as there may be a long wait before they can have more specialized help, so the importance of understanding the developmental sequences should now be clear.

We come back now to the type of assessment to be

carried out, in order that the clinician may be in a position to (a) know which children to refer for specialist help, (b) understand what sort of help is appropriate, and (c) be able to give some initial advice to parents.

Assessement of language development will be discussed in a very practical way, with a view to guiding those who are not necessarily language specialists but who are responsible for the early assessment of handicapped children in developmental clinics. The wide range of expensive tests and standardized scales which are now available will not be included in the discussion, as these are often confined to use by specialists. They are not, in any case, essential to a first assessment of a child with a language handicap. The only 'scale' we are concerned with here is the rational one of the developmental sequence of prelanguage and language development discussed in previous chapters. With this understanding as in-built equipment, the clinician should be in a good position to carry out a reliable initial assessment, sorting out those with a real problem for referral to specialists for further help.

THE STARTING-POINT

Information from referral letters, developmental history, and initial observation of the child will give some rough idea of the developmental level the child has achieved. It is not rational or feasible to start the assessment at the very earliest stages of development and work right through with each child in the short time available for the session, so this initial estimate of approximate level is important. The 'short time' referred to is not just the clinician's time, but rather the time that the child can tolerate. Most preschool children, particularly those who are retarded or handicapped, have only a limited amount of concentration to give. With an active $2\frac{1}{2}$ year old, for example, the clinician may have only about 20 minutes of possible cooperation, so it is important not to lose any of this by starting the assessment at too high or too low a level. Ideally the assessment should start just below the child's probable level, as a measure of initial success is important to the child. If, for example, the child is observed to follow simple directions but to say only two or three words, there is probably no need to start the assessment right back at the stage of direct (non-symbolic) communication and object recognition. Reports can be very misleading, however, so even a few minutes of initial observation are important. This can often be done when fetching the child from the waiting room. We should be particularly wary of reports that a child 'understands everything I say'. This could be at the stage of situational understanding (page 30) rather than true verbal comprehension. Again, this can be observed by watching and listening while the mother gets her child to leave whatever he is playing with in the waiting room and come into the examination room. Assessment starts from this very first moment of contact, and continues through every moment the child is in the room, even if he is just playing while the clinician talks to the parents.

In the following pages, assessment will be discussed stage by stage, starting at the early, prelanguage stages. This gives the overall procedure in a rational order. The initial observation and reports will give some indication of where, in this sequence, to start with each child.

ARRANGEMENT OF ROOM

This practical point may seem trivial, but it can make all the difference between success and failure with difficult children. More details of dealing with difficult children are given on page 85. There is no time to start searching for assessment material or arranging tables and chairs when the child is actually in the room, as he will need the clinician's full attention and observation all the time, so that not a moment is wasted. Cooperation with young children can easily be lost in these first few minutes if the room or the clinician are not ready. It is up to the clinician to adapt quickly to the child so that confidence is established.

It is well worth the extra few minutes it takes before fetching the child, to see that appropriately sized tables and chairs are in position, and that all necessary assessment material is readily accessible. Put on the table some toy or piece of equipment that is likely to interest the child, but avoid a clutter of material. Figure 3 shows a suitable arrangement for most preschool children who are mature enough to sit at a small table.

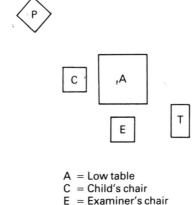

A = Low table
C = Child's chair
E = Examiner's chair
P = Parent's chair
T = Box of test material

Figure 3   Seating arrangement for assessment of pre-school child

The examiner should sit on a child-sized chair, so that he is on the same level as the child. In most cases parents should be near to, but slightly behind the child, so that they can give reassurance by their presence yet not interfere with the relationship between examiner and child. Children under three years are often best assessed at a full-sized table sitting on their mother's knee. This gives reassurance to shy children, and keeps the very active ones anchored.

Sitting down and taking coats off should not be enforced, as the assessment can quite well be carried out with the child wandering around the room; in fact this is sometimes essential (see page 90).

THE STAGES IN PRELANGUAGE DEVELOPMENT

Basic, direct communication

With very young, or very retarded children, in whom there is as yet no verbal development, it may be necessary to begin the assessment at this very basic level. This also applies to so-called 'non-communicating' children, in other words those showing autistic behaviour. There is likely to be some basic communication ability in these children, however primitive, which may have already been built into some system of 'situational' communication patterns. It is the clinician's role to assess what is already there, and advise on how this can be extended.

We need to look at receptive and expressive aspects, even at this basic level. The assessment can be carried out by observing communication between parents and child in appropriately structured situations. Parents are the people with whom the child is most likely to attempt some communication.

Receptive communication

Ask the parents to get the child to follow simple everyday directions such as to come across the room to them; to put his coat on; to bring them a toy. Watch carefully to see what aspects of the communication, if any, the child can follow. It may be necessary for the parent to go over to the child, take his hand and lead him across the room. Or the child may be able to follow the sort of total communication pattern described on p. 14, where the mother uses a combination of voice, facial expression and gross gesture, such as holding out her arms. It may be possible to reduce some of these clues and still get a response. An example of this is Arthur, a severely retarded autistic child who could only respond to unfamiliar people if his hands were actually put on the material he was required to use. His own nurse was able to call him to her, by using a familiar phrase and voice pattern, backed up by gesture with her arms. She was then asked to call him to her without the gesture, and Arthur responded appropriately. In an unfamiliar setting, with an unfamiliar person, he could only manage the most basic receptive communication of actually being taken through the activity with his hands. In a well-learnt situation, with his own nurse, he could already dispense with some of the situational clues, and come in response to the familiar voice and phrase pattern. Teaching indications with such a child are towards (a) extending the phrases to which he will respond with familiar people, but only gradually reducing the extra situational clues, and (b) extending the range of people to whom he will give this response by keeping the communication pattern constant.

Expressive communication

It is unlikely that children still at this very basic level of communication will initiate much communication with a stranger, so it is best to create a situation of 'I want', so that the child will be motivated to communicate. There is usually a toy, a sweet, a biscuit or some 'fetish' object that he particularly likes to have. This can be put just out of his reach but within his view on a table or shelf. Watch whether he (a) struggles to get it and screams with frustration, which does not rate as a communication at all; (b) takes his mother across the room and directs her hand towards it. This is a very basic and direct communication, but it is personally directed towards his mother, or whichever adult he takes; (c) holds up his hand towards it with an asking type of vocalization. This is slightly more mature, but still a 'direct' communication, in that the hand held out and vocalization form some sort of a communication pattern.

Other situations may arise during the session, when spontaneous communication can be observed. For example, a small child who was getting tired of the discussion between his parents and the clinician, got his coat and took it over to his mother – a very direct, but meaningful communication. It is important that parents understand the need to respond to these communications whenever possible, to encourage the child to continue with them, and extend his communication to other things. In the example given, there is no reason why the parent should not put the child's coat on while continuing to talk to the clinician, so that the child has at least some partial reward for his communication.

Situational understanding and situational phrase patterns (approximate age level 9 to 12 months)

Moving on to the transitional stage between direct communication and language, we need to assess the understanding and use of familiar phrase patterns where there is a good back-up of situational clues.

Once again it is best to do the assessment via the parents or other familiar adult, as they form part of the 'situation' in which the communication patterns have been learnt. Looking at receptive and expressive aspects separately, a useful assessment procedure is as follows.

Assessment of the stages in prelanguage development

Receptive situational communication patterns

Find out from the parents what phrases they commonly
use with their child in the course of daily living activities
or play, and to which ones they would expect an appropriate response. The usual ones that can be tried out
during the session are:
'Give us a kiss', when the child is appropriately seated on
his mother's knee.
'Do pat-a-cake', when seated in the usual position for this
game.
'Arms up', in preparation for dressing or undressing.
'Come here', or 'come to Mummy', when being called
from across the room.
 There are at least three developmental stages to notice
in the way the communication is received and responded
to, which the clinician should observe.

(1) The need for a massive back-up of situational clues,
including the right time and place, the right person, and
the right accompanying gestures and facial expression, as
well as the right rhythmic and tonal pattern of the phrase.
This is an early stage of transition which will need a good
deal of consolidation before it is firmly established as
situational understanding related specifically to the
phrase. This might be difficult to demonstrate in an
assessment situation, but unless the parents' reports are
very reliable, some attempt should be made to achieve an
observable response. At least the clinician can observe
how extensive the communication by the parents needs to
be by getting them to attempt to elicit a response.
(2) A response to the familiar phrase said in the usual
way by the usual person, but not necessarily in the usual
place, and with only minimal back-up clues. This can be
observed by making sure that the familiar adult uses the
phrase without additional clues other than the familiar
situation such as seating position. This child is ready for

help in moving on to the next stage of understanding the phrases themselves.

(3) An ability to respond to the familiar phrase when it is said by an unfamiliar person in an unfamiliar setting. This stage can be assessed by the clinician doing the asking, but still using the familiar phrase with the usual rhythmic and tonal pattern. This child is ready for plenty of extension of phrase patterns in daily living at home.

Expressive communication using patterned intonation

This is best observed incidentally during the course of the assessment session. This means that the clinician must be alert throughout, to pick up any indication of patterned communications. These often occur when no notice is being taken of the child, for example when the clinician is talking to the parents. The child may take a toy up to his parents to show them. Notice exactly how this is done, and what, if any, vocalization or gesture accompanies the action. If no communication occurs spontaneously, get the parents to play with the child, with the clinician sitting in the background observing. If the play material is interesting enough, and the situation fairly relaxed, this will usually elicit a sample of the child's expressive communication. Notice the following three stages:

(1) Simple 'asking' communications consisting of holding out hands accompanied by a particular tonal pattern, usually with an upward inflection. Pointing to what he wants, with or without the same tonal pattern. Pointing is a simple gesture, but it is one step beyond a 'direct' communication.

(2) Use of slightly more extended vocalization, accompanying a familiar action, such as 'ee-ar', or 'ta', on transferring an object from one person to another.

(3) Use of phrase patterns in which simulated sentences

can be recognized during play. For example, Susan, playing with the doll's house toys, picked up the toy telephone and vocalized long strings of jargon, simulating her mother's telephone voice, and ending always with 'e-yo' (hello).

These stages of prelanguage expression can be encouraged by responding appropriately whenever possible, and sometimes by supplying the appropriate phrase in response, if the child's intention is clear enough. This adult feedback should be carried out with extreme care at this stage, however, because a wrong interpretation can only confuse the child.

Assessment of object recognition (Approximate age level 12 months)

The stage of object recognition must be reached before a child can begin to learn object labels. A symbol, such as a toy model, a picture, or a word, cannot be related meaningfully to an object, as a label, until the child has an internalized concept of that object. He cannot, for example, understand the word 'chair', as related to all chairs until he has an internalized concept of a chair. He may understand the word at a 'situational' level, referred only to his own chair at specific times of day, as part of a feeding sequence, but he will not be able to point to any chair in response to 'where's the chair?'. He must first understands that all objects with the characteristics of four legs, a seat and back, intended for sitting on, belong to the same group of objects. He has then an internalized concept of the object 'chair' to which a symbol can later be attached. This is explained more fully on page 22. At this point we are concerned with how to assess this important prelanguage stage of object recognition.

Assessment is simple enough. Real objects, not toys and

pictures, must be used, and they should, as far as possible, be similar to but not identical to the ones the child is used to. If he is used to metal spoons, for example, it is best to use a metal spoon for assessment rather than a plastic one.

Three or four everyday objects should be used, either placed on the table together, or handed one by one to the child. Suitable objects are a cup, a spoon, a hairbrush, a toothbrush and a telephone. Observe whether the child demonstrates recognition of the objects by attempting to use them appropriately. At least three levels of achievement can be defined, which will give the examiner an indication of whether the child has only just reached this stage and needs plenty of consolidation, or whether his understanding of objects is well established as a basis for learning symbols. The stages to observe can be defined as follows:

(1) Object recognition just beginning. At this stage the child will recognize only one or two of the objects and may need a few extra clues to enable him to attempt appropriate use. For example his mother may need to say 'brush your hair' in order for him to demonstrate use of the brush. The objects may be related appropriately to himself, but not adaptively. For example he may put the brush to his hair, but get it the wrong way round and not really brush with it. The advice at this stage is for the mother to help the child use everyday objects at the appropriate time through daily living. Let him handle it, and help him to use it, before the adult takes over. This should be extended to all meaningful objects in regular use at home.

(2) He will pick up and use one or two of the objects appropriately and adaptively without extra clues. For example he may pick up the toothbrush, get it the right way round, and brush his teeth with it. These children

may still need some consolidation at this stage, but can also be helped on to the next stage of easy symbols (see below).

(3) If the stage of object recognition is really well established, and the child's understanding well beyond this, he may demonstrate some extension of the object's use such as brushing his mother's hair, or the examiner's hair; stirring with the spoon in the cup; picking up the telephone receiver and vocalizing jargon into it, or attempting to dial. With such children the assessment can proceed quickly on to the stages of symbolic understanding.

Older, very retarded institutionalized children will often not use the cup, spoon or brush, as these objects have become too situation-bound and uninteresting for them. They will, however, nearly always use the toothbrush and telephone if they are developmentally ready for this.

ASSESSMENT OF SYMBOLIC UNDERSTANDING
(Approximate age level 15 months to 3 years)

Large doll play (Approximately 15 to 18 months)

When object recognition is firmly established, the foundation is laid for the development of symbolic understanding. Once a child has an internalized object concept, or internalized awareness of an object class such as 'cup', 'ball', then he is ready to begin to understand that this object can be represented by something else such as a toy model, picture or word. As explained in Chapter 2 this understanding begins with recognition of representations that have many similar perceptual attributes to the actual object.

In assessment it is best to use objects that are in daily use in every household, so that there is unlikely to be the complication of failure resulting from inexperience of the actual objects. This applies, too, to the earlier stage of object recognition. Try to duplicate the objects used in the object recognition section by toy models of large doll or teddy bear size. A Wendy House teaset is useful, with the addition of a large doll, and doll's brush and comb. Give the child the doll and toy brush, at first, as this is the most usual first step in understanding. If he does not respond, demonstrate by brushing the doll's hair for him and then persuade him to do it himself. When he has achieved this, give him the doll and the cup, and repeat the procedure. If both these activities are spontaneously successful, give him a selection of the toys (such as teapot, milk jug, cup, saucer) and see whether he will act out a sequence with or without demonstration. If he plays appropriately and spontaneously at any of these stages, he is ready to move on to the next developmental stage. If he needs a demonstration and then succeeds, he is ready for learning at this stage, but not yet ready to move on. If he fails altogether, he needs more consolidation at the previous stage of experience with real objects. These stages can be summarized as follows:

(1) Uses brush and/or cup with doll only after demonstration; needs further learning at this stage.

(2) Uses brush and/or cup spontaneously; ready to move on to the next stage.

(3) Acts out simple sequences such as pouring a cup of tea and then giving the doll a drink; well established at this stage of understanding and already using the material as a 'language'; should be more than ready for higher levels of symbolic understanding.

Small doll play (Approximately 18 to 21 months)

The next stage of assessment is to see whether the child

can understand representations that are more remote (perceptually) from the objects they represent. Dolls and furniture of doll's house size are useful for this. Many of the toys, such as the small beds, bear little perceptual relationship to the child's own bed. The overall shape, or gestalt, is the same, but little else, so the child must really be able to recognize this as a symbol, which represents but is different from the real thing. There is often a transitional stage at which the child will attempt to sit on the tiny chairs, thus recognizing the gestalt, but not fully appreciating that it only has representational meaning as an object.

Give the child only three items at first, as too many could confuse him. More can be added if he seems ready for this. The suggested combinations are (a) doll, bed and blanket, (b) doll, table and chair. His understanding of these symbolic toys will be demonstrated by the way he attempts to relate them. His response will indicate whether he is just ready to understand these symbols or whether he has fully established this stage and is ready to move on to two-dimensional representations. The following two stages are suggested for observation:

(1) Relates two of the toys only. He may lie the child on the bed and fail to use the blanket, or sit the doll on the chair and fail to use the table. Demonstrate relating these toys and see whether this helps him. If so, he is learning ready at this stage.

(2) He may spontaneously relate three or more components, such as putting the doll in bed and covering it up, or seating the doll at the table and feeding it from a tiny cup. He may act out simple sequences with the toys, such as putting the doll in the bath, drying it and putting it to bed. Such a child is using the toys as a language substitute and is more than ready for more advanced levels of understanding.

Object – picture matching (Approximately 21 to 24 months)

The next stage in the development of symbolic under-standing involves the introduction of two-dimensional representations, in the form of pictures. Very clear col-oured pictures are used at first, depicting everyday objects against a plain background, so that they are perceptually clear. The Ladybird Picture Series (Wingfield, 1970) pro-vides many suitable pictures, which can be cut out and stuck on cards.

In order to find out whether a child, who has no speech and perhaps no verbal understanding, can understand and recognize pictures, we can get him to match real objects to the pictures. Real objects rather than toys are used, because at this first stage of two-dimensional under-standing he can only manage one symbol at a time. The procedure is as follows:

Put out four of the pictures. Demonstrate what is wanted by producing one of the matching objects and placing it on the appropriate picture. Leave it there, hand the child the next object and encourage him to select the right picture. When the series of four pictures has been completed in this way, with or without help from the examiner, change the order of the pictures and see if the child can do it without any demonstration. Examples of suitable picture – object pairs are a spoon, cup, brush and bunch of keys.

When possible the object and pictorial representation should be different colours, so as to make sure that the child is really matching object and symbol, and not a simple colour match. He might, for example, match a pink brush to a picture of a pink brush, but fail when the picture is of a white brush. This is deviant, as colour matching usually comes later in development, but then these are deviant children, and we need to be sure just what sort of understanding is being demonstrated.

If the child names the picture or object to help the match, then he is probably well ahead of this stage in language development, but avoid naming it for him. The stages to watch for are as follows:

(1) Just manages one or two correctly, after plenty of preliminary help. This child needs plenty of consolidation at this level before moving on to the next stage.

(2) Succeeds without help the second time round, once he understands the task after initial demonstration. This child is ready to move on to the next stage.

(3) Succeeds easily and at once, perhaps with some spontaneous naming of the objects or pictures. This child is developmentally well beyond this stage.

Toy – picture matching (Approximately 24 to 27 months)

In asking a child to match a toy representation of an object to a pictorial representation of the same object, one is asking him to match one type of symbol to another. This is clearly a more advanced stage in the understanding and use of symbols than when only one type of symbol is being used. As with object – picture matching, the material should be selected in such a way that there is no possibility of a match by some single attribute such as colour or size, which might avoid the interpretation of the symbol. For example if the picture of the cup is the biggest picture, the toy cup should not be the biggest toy; or if the cup in the picture is blue, the toy cup should be some other colour. In this way the examiner can be sure that the match is via the *object* concept, as illustrated on Figure 4.

This is a relatively advanced stage in the understanding and use of non-verbal symbols. If there is no verbal language at all by the time a child reaches this stage, something is already out of step. There certainly should be

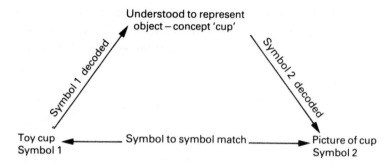

Figure 4   The processes involved in matching toys to pictures

some understanding of verbal labels even if there is no expressive language.

The assessment procedure is the same as for object – picture matching, including demonstrations when necessary. The amount of help a child needs to learn the task is part of the assessment, and indicates whether he is (a) not ready for learning at this stage, (b) ready for learning at this stage, or (c) well established at this stage. These stages of readiness can be checked by observation, as with object – picture matching.

Gesture – picture matching (Approximately 2½ to 3 years)

Some handicapped children, particularly deaf children, may need assessment at this more advanced level of symbol–symbol matching. Non-handicapped children often find this sort of task confusing, because it is much easier for them to match the word to the picture.

With children who have no language, it is a useful stage to assess because it can be broken down into receptive and expressive aspects, and give valuable information as to whether a non-verbal language such as signing would help the child. The verbal language equivalent would be selecting objects by use (receptive language); and telling the use of objects (expressive language). This is clearly a more advanced stage of language usage (verbal and non-verbal) than matching two types of symbol, whether this is selecting objects in response to naming (object–word matching) or matching a toy to a picture.

Pictures need to be carefully selected so that a gesture representing their use is clear. Suitable examples are (a) cup matched with drinking gesture; (b) hairbrush matched with brushing gesture; (c) teapot matched with pouring gesture; and (d) car matched with driving gesture. The procedure is as follows:

Receptive gesture language

Put out the four pictures in front of the child. Give him a clear gesture, and indicate that you want him to select the appropriate picture. Give as much help as necessary, because this is part of the assessment. He may need to have the whole set demonstrated before he understands what is wanted if he is not used to gesture. In this case it is advisable to give a second set of pictures to see whether the learning carries over.

Expressive gesture language

This should be done after the receptive assessment as most children will need to learn the gesture before they can use it. Point to one picture at a time and indicate to the child that you want him to give the gesture. Again, give as much help as needed for him to learn the task. If all the pictures have to be demonstrated first, use a second set to see if the learning has carried over.

Chapter 6

ASSESSMENT OF THE STAGES IN VERBAL LANGUAGE DEVELOPMENT

THE FIRST VERBAL LABEL (Approximate age level 18–21 months)

When the child reaches the stage of his first true word, used or understood as a symbol, he has probably already achieved a fund of 'situational' phrases to which he can respond appropriately, and he has achieved the stage at which he can understand that a symbol can stand for or represent an object or person. The first word, used or understood as a verbal label, may occur during the later stages of the development of symbolic understanding, perhaps overlapping in time with the development of his understanding of pictures.

The gradual development from situational understanding to one of the earliest verbal labels can be exemplified by the word 'mum', 'mummy', or 'mamma'. At first the sound 'mum-mum' occurs during states of 'I want', when the child needs attention; this becomes more situationally specific so that it occurs only in situations where the need is usually supplied by the mother, such as hunger or discomfort from a soiled nappie. The word next becomes generalised to any adult female, and finally to his mother as a specific person represented by a specific verbal label. In assessment, it is important to find out, by close questioning of the parents and by observation of the child, which of these stages a child has reached in connection with any reported verbal label. The procedure for assessing the first verbal labels is as follows.

Find out from the parents what words the child is thought to understand at this level, and try to demonstrate a selective response. An example is demonstrated in the film 'Helping Language Development' (Cooper Moodley and Reynell, 1978). Fiona is still mainly at the stage of situational understanding, but when the speech therapist says 'Oh you're not listening, Mummy's listening', Fiona turns round to look at her mother, thus demonstrating that the word 'Mummy' is understood as a verbal symbol specifically related to her mother. If the child is reported to understand the word 'teddy', or 'spoon', get the mother to ask for it and see whether the child looks at the object named. At this early stage the child is more likely to respond to his mother's voice than to the examiner's.

Once the understanding of verbal labels has begun, the comprehension vocabulary should expand fairly rapidly. Expressive language follows a few months later, but at this early stage it is more important to assess verbal comprehension.

SELECTION OF COMMON OBJECTS IN RESPONSE TO NAMING (Approximate age level 1½ to 2 years)

If a child can select a few familiar objects in response to naming, he has really achieved the first step in verbal language as a system of symbols, beyond the stage of symbolic understanding. This is an important stage to assess, and the procedure is as follows.

Use real objects, not toys or pictures, so that the child is relating a word to an object and not to another type of symbol, which is more difficult. Suitable common objects are the same ones that are used in previous stages for object recognition, namely a cup, a brush, a spoon, a ball, a shoe or a sock. Put four of the objects in front of the child and see whether he will select the named object in response to 'where's the . . .'. He may pick it up or just give a selective glance. Whatever type of response he gives should be quickly reinforced with praise and encouragement, to give him confidence for further responses. Care must be taken to ensure that the selective response is to the word and to no other clue such as an inadvertent gesture on the part of the parents, or even the examiner looking at the object named. Handicapped children are sometimes very quick to pick up these unintentional non-verbal clues. For the same reason, the objects should not be asked for in the order in which they lie on the table, and do not, of course, ask for an object that the child is already handling or playing with. It will be necessary to get the child's full attention, even if this is only possible momentarily, before each request is made. With some children it will be necessary, too, to help them scan the objects before asking the question, to make sure they have seen all four objects. By careful control of the child's attention, careful timing of the questions, and careful observation of the responses, it should be possible to have a clear indication of whether the child has reached one of the following stages:

(1) Does not understand the object labels, although he can follow the situational phrase 'give me the . . .' or 'where is the . . .' by handing whichever object is nearest.

(2) Selects one or two of the objects correctly but not always consistently.

(3) A clear and reliable selective response.

WORD COMBINATIONS (Approximate age level 2 to $2\frac{1}{4}$ years)

It is more important to assess the understanding of word

combinations than to elicit these in expressive language, although both are important. Once a child can assimilate and relate two 'operative' words, he has reached this level of development in terms of central language. The use of word combinations in expressive language is likely to follow fairly soon after this. Children who have specific expressive difficulties may be held up for some time at this stage, but provided the comprehension is there, they can usually make themselves understood by a combination of single words and gesture. A delay in comprehension at this stage is serious, and needs plenty of intensive work, as this is the basis of understanding sentences, and the root for taking language beyond the naming stage.

In assessment of verbal comprehension at this stage it is best to use simple object labels that you know the child understands. This should have become clear from the previous section. The question now is whether he can assimilate two at once and relate them appropriately. Choose the most obvious relationship, such as 'put the spoon in the box', 'put teddy on the table', as the child is not expected to understand prepositions yet. He is simply required to select the two objects named and relate them in the obvious way. There must, of course, be a choice of at least four objects to select from, and it is best to have five or six if the child can manage this in terms of perceptual span. Toys or real objects can be used, as by this stage toy representations are meaningful as symbols. The following sets are examples of real objects or toys which can be used. It is best not to mix objects and toys in the same set.

Objects: brush, cup, spoon, box, plate, fork.
Examples of directions using this set are: 'put the spoon in the cup', 'put the cup on the plate'.

It is important to give the directions in such a way that

78

both objects are named before the child picks up one of them, so that it is truly an assimilation of two named objects. Children who have not reached this stage of understanding typically pick up only one of the named objects.

Learning stages to watch for are as follows.

(1) Child fails completely or selects only one of the pair, even after some help has been given. Such a child is not yet ready for this stage of learning and needs further consolidation at the previous stage.

(2) Child manages at least one pair correctly and more when some help is given. This child is ready for plenty of teaching at this stage of understanding.

(3) Child succeeds in all requests (at least three pairs should be asked for) without help. This child has achieved this stage of development and is ready to move on.

Expressive aspects of word combinations

Without a good deal of experience it is sometimes difficult to elicit word combinations deliberately, but most children who are able to do this will produce at least one word combination during the session, perhaps in free play with small toys. The examiner should be alert to observe and record any such word combinations and check these against the parents' reports. The utterances can only be assessed as true word combinations if there is a definite bringing together of two words, not learnt as a whole phrase. Thus, one would discount 'little boy', 'pretty flower' etc. but include 'where Mummy?', 'Daddy gone', 'ee-ar lady' etc. These early expressive word combinations rarely include two object labels, but usually are the name of a person or single object combined with a 'situational' word or phrase, as in the examples given above.

NOUN–VERB STAGE (Approximate age level $2\frac{1}{2}$–$2\frac{3}{4}$ years)

As explained on page 35 this is a more difficult stage than that of relating two named objects or uttering word combinations, even though it is still a stage of only two 'operative' words, and perhaps only two-word sentences. A definite action word is more difficult for a child to understand than an object label or 'situational' word, because perceptual aid is less clear. Assessment of the understanding of action words or concepts is most easily arranged by getting the children to select objects or toys by use. This usually means that they only need to assimilate one word, but it is at the noun–verb level of understanding, where the subject is implied. This stage is sometimes assessed by using pictures, such as 'show me the girl running', '. . . the boy sleeping'. In a detailed analysis of language this more sophisticated type of assessment is clearly essential, but from the point of view of the clinician in a developmental clinic, the essential basic understanding at this stage of action words can be assessed by using the objects or toys as in previous sections and asking questions such as 'which one do we sit on?', 'which one do we sleep in', 'which one do we pour the tea from?'. There should be a choice of at least four objects or toys. Learning readiness can be assessed by observing the following types of response.

(1) No understanding without massive situational clues. The child may need a back-up of familiar phrases to supplement the question, or he may only respond in familar situations. Parents often supply the necessary clues without being asked, in a test situation. For example if the question was 'which one do we sleep in?', the mother may expand this by saying 'where do you go bye-byes, and Mummy kiss you goodnight?' etc. Such a

child has not yet achieved learning readiness at this stage and needs further work at earlier levels.

(2) Child selects a few of the objects or toys correctly but not all. He is ready for plenty of help at this stage of understanding, in both play and daily living.

(3) Child responds easily without hesitation or error. This child is ready for higher levels of understanding.

Expressive language

Simple noun–verb sentences may occur spontaneously during the session, but if in any doubt, the clinician can elicit these in play situations. This is done by carrying out some simple action with the toys and asking an open-ended question such as 'what happened?', 'what did I do?'. Examples of simple actions which interest children, and which will usually produce an appropriate response from children who are at this level are.

(1) Run two toy cars into each other, or run one into a doll.
(2) Put a doll on a chair and then tip it off.
(3) Build a tower of bricks and knock it down.

Notice whether the child uses only the verb, such as 'falled down', or whether he produces a true noun-verb sentence such as 'boy fall down', or 'falled off chair'. This will indicate whether he is learning ready, or stabilised at this stage of expressive language.

RELATING THREE OR MORE 'OPERATIVE' WORDS, AND USE OF SIMPLE SENTENCES (Approximate age level $2\frac{1}{2}$–$3\frac{1}{2}$ years)

The exact developmental level at which this stage is achieved will of course depend on the particular type of sentences used and the complexity of ideas they represent. For a more detailed assessment the examiner would have to use one of the standardized assessment scales, but for the purpose of the developmental clinician, a rough guide as to whether or not the child is within the normal range can be achieved without these more sophisticated tools. In the following directions, which include three or more 'operative' words, children need to understand words that relate to more abstract concepts than nouns and verbs, as explained on page 36. The way in which the assessment of verbal comprehension is carried out, at this level of understanding, must depend on the ingenuity of the clinician in constructing simple requests, and on the material available. The requests must be such that the child needs to understand more than simple two-word combinations to follow the directions, and this is most easily done by introducing prepositions and/or adjectives. Examples, using simple material, which can give some guidance to the clinician are: 'put the *spoon* and the *cup* in the *box*'; 'put the *red brick* in the *tin*'; 'find the *biggest brick* and give it to *Mummy*'.

Expressive aspects a word combinations

Assessment of the child's ability to use simple sentences will be carried out in the same way as with word combinations and noun–verb combinations as explained above. Sentences may be heard in spontaneous conversation, or elicited through play situations with 'what happened?', 'what did I do?' requests (see above). Parents' reports are useful with shy children, but should be checked if at all possible with observations during the session.

ASSESSMENT OF HIGHER LEVELS OF LANGUAGE UNDERSTANDING AND USE

If preschool children have already reached these more advanced stages of language development, it is unlikely that they still have major problems with central language. There can be specific and persisting problems, however, which continue into school age. The detailed investigations which these need is not often appropriate in a first assessment at a developmental clinic, but requires a more specialized approach, which is beyond the scope of this book. At this level of a central language, where the child can use and understand more complex sentences, the problems evident in the clinic, if any, are likely to be more concerned with intelligibility and articulation. As a rough guide, intelligibility can be rated by the clinician at one of the following three levels:

(1) Unintelligible except possibly to his parents, even when the context is known. This child clearly needs specialist help, or he will encounter enormous frustrations socially, however good his actual central language.

(2) Intelligible only if the context is known. In describing a picture, for example, or a scene enacted with toys, it may be clear what he is trying to say, as the possible range is circumscribed by the situation, but it may still be virtually impossible to understand spontaneous utterances when the context is not so circumscribed. This is a very common situation in older children with a persisting language handicap, and needs help.

(3) Intelligible but with minor deviances in articulation affecting certain sounds such as 's' or 'r'. This is much less serious, and further referral will depend on other things such as social awareness of the difficulty and central language level. Direct work on tidying up minor articulation difficulties is best deferred until the child has a central

language age of at least 4½ years, otherwise a focus on specific speech sounds may interfere with the language development.

CONCLUSION

The procedures described above should enable clinicians to assess the approximate developmental level of a child's language and communication, and to enable him to select those children who have a real problem needing specialist help. The emphasis has been put on the early stages of language development, including prelanguage (see Chapter 5), rather than on the more sophisticated type of assessment needed for older children who have a very specific and persistent language handicap. These older children (5+ years) will usually have been picked up at an earlier stage and some help already provided. It is the younger children for whom the developmental clinician often has the responsibility of the first assessment, and who needs to make the decision as to whether further help is needed at that stage. Another reason for concentrating on the early stages is that recent research has shown that great progress can be made with young children referred in the early stages of a language handicap (see Chapter 10) and perhaps saved from greater problems later on. A specific central language handicap may become evident between the ages of 2 and 3 years, and appropriate help at this age can often enable the child to overcome most of the difficulty by school age.

Chapter 7

ASSESSMENT OF DIFFICULT CHILDREN

The procedures, as described in chapters 5 and 6 above, are suitable for the large majority of young children, or older mentally handicapped children. There are a few children, however, sometimes described as 'untestable', who may need special modifications and special techniques of handling, although the basic assessment stages described here can still be applied. In the author's opinion, the word 'untestable' should never be used. It is an admission of failure to adapt on the part of the examiner. Certainly there are many young, and/or handicapped children who do not respond to specific test items presented in a specific way, but there is no child who cannot be 'assessed' provided the procedures are adapted to the child, and the standards used are based on an understanding of child development rather than on rigid test scores. The procedures described here should allow plenty of flexibility, with opportunities for different forms of presentation adapted to the child. The question to be answered is, what stage of development has the child reached in terms of language and communication, is this consistent with his age, or does it need specific help? If a child does not respond to a particular item presented in the usual way, then it is up to the clinician to understand the situation and assess the same stage of development by suitable modification of the usual procedures.

It is often said that some people are 'good' with children, and some are not blessed with this specific 'gift'. What does this mean? To be 'good' with children, or to 'have a way with children' simply means to be sensitive to the child, and to adapt quickly to that child. Some people do have a greater sensitivity to children than others, but in everyone this comes to a greater or lesser degree with experience and observation of children. There are clear techniques in handling certain types of difficult behaviour that can be learnt. No one should despair that he or she cannot manage difficult or very young children in an assessment situation, if this is understood as a sensitivity to the child, adaptation to the child, and adoption of certain techniques of approach. (Any clinician who is completely confident in handling all types of non-responsive or difficult children in a clinic situation will probably want to miss out this chapter. It is intended to give some guidance and understanding to those who encounter difficulties and would welcome some hints on specific techniques to use. Each child is a unique individual, so the guidance can only be given in a general way, with examples of some of the extremes of behaviour.)

VERY SHY, WITHDRAWN CHILDREN

This is not uncommon among 2–4-year-old children, when they encounter unfamiliar situations such as coming to the clinic. Some degree of initial shyness is, of course, expected. It is unusual for a child to show no initial wariness at all, and to be equally responsive to a stranger as to familiar adults. This normal range of shyness is easily overcome by the child's interest in the assessment material, and some initial success in what he is asked to do. The old idea of 'establishing rapport' with a child before starting the assessment is not advised with young children. There is nothing so shy-making as a direct confrontation with an adult trying to 'establish rapport' by making conversation. The direction should be away from this direct personal approach, and focus on something less threatening to the child such as toys or interesting test material. If his attention is directed straight away towards this concrete material, with the examiner observing but not immediately interacting, the child will quickly relax. There are those excessively shy children, however, who come into the room hiding behind their mother's skirt, and who cover their faces and retreat if a stranger so much as looks at them. The answer to this is not to 'look at' them. This is done by seating the child on his mother's knee, with a shoebox full of interesting small toys on the table in front of him, and getting the mother to play naturally with her child. The examiner sits behind the child, some distance away, and observes by using peripheral vision while apparently writing or reading. This gives an opportunity to note down observations while appearing not to be watching the child. If the child looks round, he should not encounter an intent stare from the examiner, but see someone quietly writing and taking no notice of him. A one-way screen is of course ideal for those who are lucky enough to have one in the clinic, but this is rare. Self-effacement by sitting well behind the child is very effective. The assessment can proceed by observation in this way for as long as the child needs it. If suitable toys are provided, symbolic understanding can be observed. Some verbal comprehension and perhaps expressive communications can also be observed by noting the interchange between mother and child. Usually it is possible for the examiner gradually to draw up to the table and join in the activity, gradually taking over the communication and so structuring the situation for different levels of assessment. It may be necessary to conduct the whole session via the mother, but a perfectly adequate assessment is possible in this way, by giving the mother *sotto voce* directions. Siblings can sometimes help, too, to relax these very shy children. Sometimes a brother or sister sitting at a small table with the handicapped child, and playing together, can help a child to lose his shyness. The examiner can assess the handicapped child by including the sibling in everything that is done.

Provided it is understood that, with these excessively shy children, it is the stranger who is the 'threat', ways can be found by which this 'threat' can be minimized by self-effacement of the examiner.

More difficult are the children whose 'shy' act is really a bid for attention. The main thing with these children is not to reinforce the behaviour by rewarding with a lot of coaxing. An indirect approach, as suggested above, is probably the best one with these children too.

RESTLESS, HYPERACTIVE CHILDREN

In contrast to the very shy children who come into the room reluctantly and are slow to get going, there are children who rush into the room and snatch at anything that takes their fancy, often ignoring any adults present and indifferent to any attempts at direct control. With such children it is particularly important to have the room carefully prepared beforehand. It is often useless, and indeed sometimes undesirable to spend time trying to quieten the child down before beginning. This can lead to frustration and perhaps precipitate a temper tantrum, and then all cooperation is lost. It is better to canalize the activity into directions that can be used for the assessment. These children are usually at a very immature stage in attention control (see page 45) such that they flit quickly from one thing to another. The examiner can use this switching of attention provided he is always ready to anticipate the child's next move. See that there is something interesting to him, and relevant to the assessment, for him to switch his attention to when the moment is right, and be ready to change onto something else before his attention is completely lost. These are exhausting children to test, but an adequate assessment can be achieved by carefully structuring the situation in this way. A suggested procedure is as follows.

Before the child comes into the room, see that all is arranged so that the examiner, but not the child, has easy access to such test material as he will need. Arrange the seating so that the child can sit on the mother's knee, even if he will only do this for short spells at a time. It is more likely to 'anchor' him momentarily than sitting on his own at a small table. A suggested arrangement is shown in Figure 5.

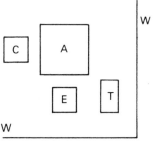

A = Full sized table
C = Child seated on parent's lap
E = Examiner
T = Box of test material
W = Walls of room

Figure 5   Seating arrangement for assessing restless, hyperactive children

A corner of the room is used so that the child cannot help himself from the box of test materials, but so that he can have breaks for roaming round the room, if necessary, without hurting himself or anything else.

Having arranged the room, the examiner puts some interesting piece of test material, suitable for the level he intends to assess, on the table where the child is to sit. The session is started with the child on the mother's knee, provided this does not meet too much resistance from the child. It is best to get through as much of the assessment as possible before he struggles to get down. This means a quick turnover of test materials, with no gaps. If there has to be a gap, for writing notes or searching for a piece of equipment, have a 'fidget toy' available to give the child; a small spinning toy is useful for this purpose. He will probably need several spells of getting down and roaming round the room. This should be allowed, and will enable the examiner to catch up with a few notes and rearrangement of test material. The assessment should be quick, but the examiner should not allow himself to be hurried. Make full use of the moments of attention the child is able to give, but do not force it to the point of frustration.

If the child will not sit down, even momentarily, and refuses even to come to the table, then the assessment must be carried out by observation, calling his attention from time to time to whatever material you want him to use. In this way it is possible to make use of his fleeting attention, by distracting him *towards* what you want him to do.

A great deal of help can be gained by checking his behaviour and achievements with the parents' expectations – 'Has he done what you would have expected?' If not, find out how they think he should have done better, and try this by restructuring the situation. They usually say that the behaviour demonstrated was fairly typical, because these children are not often particularly sensitive to new environments, and unfamiliarity does not alter their behaviour in the same way that it does with very shy children.

SELF-DETERMINED, NON-COOPERATING CHILDREN

It is common for children in the 2 to 3 year range to be unable to adapt to what an adult wants them to do, but to be interested enough in the test material to become absorbed in their own choice of activity. This sort of behaviour may be exaggerated in some very determined children, and persist beyond the usual age range. Assessment with such children will only be successful if the clinician is resourceful enough (a) to make full use of what the child chooses to do, by using it as the assessment focus, and (b) to manipulate the situation and presentation of material so that the child 'chooses' to do what is wanted. Typically these children, if boys, will become fixated on toy cars. It is best, therefore, not to produce these until towards the end of the session. If a child does find one early in the session, or brings one in with him, this can sometimes be used as a 'reward'. The car is put on the table within the child's range of vision, but not within his reach, and is given to him immediately for a short play at the end of each test item. Again, if cars are the only things that interest him, introduce verbal directions related to the cars so that the stages of verbal comprehension and expressive language can be carried out with the cars as a focus – for example 'where is the car?', 'here is the garage, put the car in the garage', 'put the green car in the garage', 'put the car and the lorry in the garage', etc. The child's level of understanding can be assessed by carefully structuring the verbal directions for different levels of understanding as in the above examples.

For expressive language, sentences may be elicited in play with the cars, for example, running one car into another – 'what happened?'.

Symbolic play can be observed by seeing whether the child can include dolls, toy trees, toy houses etc. in his play, or whether he is content just to push a car along saying 'brrm-brrm'.

A similar technique can be used to build the assessment around the child's choice of activity at all levels.

A direct confrontation, or insistence on a certain type of activity should be avoided with such children. They will not give way, and this can only lead to extreme frustration and a breakdown of all possible cooperation. Taking a toy away from the child against his will, for example, is not advised with this type of child. At the same time, it must be the clinician who is in command and who directs operations in a subtle way so that the child is led along through the assessment stages without realizing it is not his own 'choice'. If he does realize this, it may lead to refusals, so tactics must be changed. In extreme cases, where children are negative and oppositional, it may be necessary to present the tests in such a way that the child does what he thinks he is being asked *not* to do. This is a tedious and exhausting way of testing which fortunately is rarely necessary.

As explained on page 46, the children who are developmentally at level 2 in attention control, often present with this self-determined, 'obstinate' type of behaviour. The clinician should understand that this is not because the child will not cooperate, but rather because he cannot. It is part of the assessment to understand his level of attention control and to use it in the assessment.

CHILDREN WITH SEVERE MOTOR DIFFICULTIES

Children who have severe motor handicaps due to cerebral palsy, often suffer an interference with speech production as a result of inadequate control of the speech musculature. It is particularly important with such children to assess their central language ability, especially verbal comprehension. This will give valuable guidance as to how far, and at what level other communication systems can be taught. Children who have passed the stage of situational understanding, and who have some understanding of symbols, can usually be taught simple head movements to indicate 'yes' and 'no', or if there is no head control, perhaps there is some other minimal movement they can make. It is surprising how much useful communication can be built up using just a 'yes–no' response. If the child has reached the stage of understanding object labels, the gesture system can be extended still further to include most of the daily needs. If the child has a really good understanding of language he is ready to be taught more sophisticated systems of communication such as communication boards, where he spells out the message at first with pictures, and then with words. Many severely handicapped children do not reach this level of verbal understanding, however, and attempts to teach them beyond their level can only lead to frustration and disappointment. Better to assess their true level and build on that.

Assessment of verbal comprehension is best carried out by using an eye-pointing response. This simply means indicating the selective response by looking at the object, or 'pointing with the eyes'. With children who have good eye control, there is usually a brief scanning of all objects, followed by fixation of the one selected. The examiner should be quick to reinforce the response with praise, so that the child knows there is communication. On the other hand, care must be taken not to arrest the scanning at the appropriate object by a too early interjection of 'good' or other reinforcement, otherwise the child may learn to scan until the selection is made for him by the examiner. Some children will just fixate the object, others may fixate and smile, or fixate and attempt to point with the arm. If eye control is not good, it is wise to have a practice period with a few easy objects first, so that the examiner may learn what constitutes a true response for that particular child. The material should be set out so that it is all within the child's perceptual range, and yet spaced so that a clear eye-pointing selection can be seen. It should be remembered that scanning may be difficult, or the range limited, in children with muscular problems, or with possible visual field restrictions.

At the stage of situational understanding, some familiar phrase may elicit a change in facial expression, an excited response, or a specific learnt movement within the child's range.

Interest shown in doll-play carried out by the examiner may indicate understanding, and some children may even direct operations by using eye-pointing. Object–picture matching and picture–toy matching can be carried out by using eye-pointing, as can all the stages of verbal comprehension.

Chapter 8

THE QUESTION OF REFERRING CHILDREN FOR ONGOING HELP

Having carried out the initial assessment, the clinician is faced with the decision as to which children have a real problem needing further referral; which children need to be kept under review for possible problems; and which children are developing within the normal range. The fact that the child has presented at the clinic at all with a language difficulty, alerts the clinician to possible problems needing further help, but these are sometimes minor and transient difficulties that can be helped by immediate advice to the parents. Care should be taken not to miss a real problem, but at the same time the resources for ongoing help are not infinite, and should be focused on those in real need. This initial assessment then, is very important, and carries a heavy weight of responsibility. Some guidance follows as to indications of a need for further referral, and the sort of help to seek. The availability of appropriate ongoing help varies greatly from one area to another, so guidance can only be given in rather general terms. In discussing children who need ongoing help, consideration is given to age, type and degree of language handicap, associated handicaps, home circumstances, and availability of help.

CONSIDERATION OF AGE

In general terms, if help is to be effective, the guiding principle is the earlier the better, from the age of 2 years onwards. Before the age of two years it is unrealistic to postulate a specific language handicap, as this is in any case only the early normal stages of language development. There may be more general developmental problems earlier than this, however, affecting behaviour, communication, and other aspects of intellectual development; such early problems could be evident in mentally handicapped or autistic children. In such cases advice can be given on helping communication at whatever developmental stage the child has reached. From the age of 2 years, early stages of more specific language handicaps may be recognized. If this is suspected, the child should be kept under careful review, and referred further if the problem has really become evident by $2\frac{1}{2}$ years.

The old idea of waiting until a child is four years old, or worse still, until he starts school, is no longer held. It has been well established that early help is feasible and effective, and should be given to any child in need as soon as possible.

Many parents do not recognize a language delay until their child is $3\frac{1}{2}$ to 4 years old, so it is common for such children to be seen for the first time at a clinic at this age. These children need help without delay if they are to catch up to near their age level by the time they start school.

DEGREE OF LANGUAGE HANDICAP

When is a language delay serious enough to amount to a handicap needing further help? Clearly it is not feasible to refer all 2 year olds, for example, who show some slight delay in talking, as this will overload the resources with children who may not have a real problem.

In general, any child whose language development is clearly out of step with his chronological age should be investigated further. Some of these children will prove to be generally retarded, the language delay being part of a general intellectual delay; but there will be others who are not intellectually retarded, who have a specific delay in one or more aspects of language development.

If a child understands no verbal labels by the age of 2 years, or has no words at all by that age, the clinician should be alerted to possible problems. If, by the age of $2\frac{1}{2}$ years, a child cannot select objects, toys or pictures in response to naming, and is not using any word combinations, that child needs help.

Approximate age levels have been given for the various developmental stages in the previous three chapters on assessment, so this should give some guidance to the clinician as to the degree of language delay, from the prelanguage stages through to the early stages of verbal language development. If a significant delay is evident at 2 years, and is still persisting at $2\frac{1}{2}$ years, the child should be referred for further help. Any child over the age of $2\frac{1}{2}$ years, showing a significant delay in receptive and/or expressive language development should be referred for further help.

It is not advisable, in a volume such as this, to try to be too exact in terms of the degree of language handicap regarded as 'significant'. This will depend on other things as well. For example, a delay in receptive language is more serious than a delay in expressive language in the early stages. Consideration should also be given to the presence or absence of other handicaps, or extensions of the language handicap, and to the availability of resources. This will all need to be weighed up in deciding on the need for further referral. However, an early language handicap should never be neglected, so when in doubt it is best to refer for further help.

TYPE OF LANGUAGE HANDICAP

General intellectual retardation

Children who have a delay in language development as part of a generalized intellectual retardation need early help, but not specifically for their language development. Parents need ongoing advice and guidance in helping their young child at home so that he can make the best use of such ability as he has in early learning and development. An approach should be made to the local educational psychologist who will be in a position to instigate whatever early educational provision may be available for such children. This may be guidance to parents at home, or, in some cases, special preschool classes.

Specific language delay affecting all aspects of language

It is common in the early stages of a developmental language handicap for verbal comprehension and expressive language both to be delayed as compared to non-verbal abilities. There are also likely to be problems of attention control and associated listening difficulties. These children need help as early as possible, with a focus on attention control and verbal comprehension. Research has shown that they respond very well to this early help, either via the parents at home, under the direction of a speech therapist, or, if they are mature enough, in a special class. For children in this category who are under school age, the best type of help is for the speech therapist to give guidance to the parents in helping the child's language through daily living at home. In that way the child may receive appropriate ongoing help all the time.

Weekly sessions of more direct speech therapy are less effective, as there is little carry over from week to week, and the sessions are separated from daily living (see Chapter 10). If there is a suitable preschool class available, and the child is emotionally ready for this, he can be helped in this group situation from $3\frac{1}{2}$ to 5 years. Such provision is, however, rare at the present time, so it may be appropriate for these children, too, to have help via the parents at home. This sort of help can be sought by referral to the local speech therapy services. It is important that parents should have ongoing advice and guidance even if there is a suitable preschool class available, as the child spends more of his daily life at home than in the class, and there should be a carry-over of help.

Specific language delay affecting only expressive language

Provided the child has a good understanding of verbal language, consistent with his age, an early delay in expressive language is less severe. A mild expressive language delay, especially in retarded children, often catches up spontaneously by $2\frac{1}{2}$ to 3 years. This is not to say, however, that such a delay should be neglected, for two reasons, (a) it may indicate the beginnings of a real language problem that needs help, and (b) if an expressive language delay persists, it can have the effect of slowing down the development of 'central' language and verbal comprehension. Any child showing a significant and specific language delay, persisting until $2\frac{1}{2}$ or 3 years, should have help. Early referral to a speech therapist is advised for such children, so that help may be given in the same way as described above. It is strongly advised that such help, with very young children, should focus on verbal comprehension as well as on expressive language, even if the verbal comprehension initially presents at an age-appropriate level. Experience has shown that verbal comprehension may suffer subsequently if the whole focus is on expressive language at the preschool stage. The position may be different with older children who have a fully established understanding of language but a persisting specific expressive handicap.

Problems of articulation and intelligibility

If this is really the only aspect of language showing difficulty or delay, these children are not usually a priority for very early help. It is generally accepted now that it is more important to establish full developmental maturity in the more central aspects of language than to focus on the production of specific speech sounds. A distinction should be made, however, between (a) immature articulation, (b) deviant coding of sounds in words, such as consonant substitutions, and (c) an inability to produce certain speech sounds; (a) and (b) are aspects of a central language difficulty, whereas (c) is more likely to have a more peripheral cause. Children in the first two categories are likely to have some central language problem which may or may not be largely resolved, apart from the problem of intelligibility. The usual pattern of recovery from a developmental language handicap is for verbal comprehension to recover first; then the more central aspects of expressive language, such as, vocabulary, sentence construction and content; and finally the appropriate coding of sounds in words. All serious problems of intelligibility, persisting after the age of $3\frac{1}{2}$ years, should be referred to a speech therapist even if other aspects of language are entirely normal, and earlier if a more extensive language handicap is suspected.

If there are known physical reasons for the difficulty, such as cerebral palsy, speech therapists can often help, at an early age, with associated feeding and drooling problems, and, if appropriate, initiate some alternative means of communication, so early referral is recommended. It is the milder cases, those that are intelligible and have normal language, but need to tidy up their articulation, that can safely wait until the age of 4 or 4½ years, by which time their central language development should have been established.

Problems of fluency

Stammering and stuttering in young children seems to be becoming less common, as a primary handicap. More often it occurs in mild form, as a transient stage during recovery from a central language handicap. In those rare cases where there is a real fluency problem in a young child, help should be sought without delay. A speech therapist will be able to advise on whether or not ongoing help is needed.

Extensive communication problems

Children presenting with these global and extensive problems, of autistic type, are usually recognized as handicapped from an early age, and there are often associated handicaps already under the supervision of a paediatrician. If this is not the case, however, paediatric referral is advised. Early educational help can be sought via the educational psychologist, as in the case of children whose language delay is due to a general intellectual delay.

CONCLUSION

To come finally to more general principles: all children who are not developing normally need help, especially those in whom the handicap affects communication. Resources for specific ongoing help are limited, so there must be someone who takes the initial responsibility of sorting out the order of priority. This responsibility often falls to the developmental clinician, and it is with this in mind that some attempt at guidance in selection has been made in this chapter. There will still be those, however, who do not have a serious enough problem to be considered a priority for referral, and yet who could benefit from help by guidance to their parents. It is also part of the developmental clinician's role, therefore, to understand enough about early language development to be able to give such ongoing advice to parents. This volume has been produced in an attempt to help with this understanding, but it is only a starting-point. Further reading is recommended, and some suggestions are listed in Appendix II.

Chapter 9

CASE STUDIES

The case studies in this chapter have been selected in order to illustrate some of the developmental patterns of language as it occurs in children with different types of handicap. There are, of course, as many individual variations within each handicap group as there are in the normal population, but there are certain general trends specific to each group described which may differ from the usual pattern. In assessing children with different handicaps who may also have developmental language problems, it is important to be aware of these group trends so that the child may be compared with others similarly handicapped rather than with non-handicapped children. Blind children, for example, develop language in a different way and at a different pace because the language–object link is more difficult for them; deaf children have an obvious difficulty in learning spoken language in the usual way and at the usual time. These general trends, and the reasons for them, are discussed briefly with each case history.

A DEAF CHILD: MARK

Mark was first seen at the assessment centre at the age of 2 years. A hearing impairment had been suspected at the age of 6 months, and was confirmed later at an audiological centre. He was classified as severely deaf, with a bilateral hearing loss of 90 db.

He was referred to the assessment centre for investigation of delayed locomotor development. Neither his medical history nor the paediatric examination revealed any neurological or muscular cause for this. He was a large, sturdy child whose locomotor development later caught up to the usual levels.

His non-verbal performance intelligence was within the average range at each assessment, but he had some initial difficulty with early symbolic understanding as well as the more obvious difficulty of verbal language learning. This early difficulty with symbols had resolved by the time he was seen at 4 years old, and non-verbal symbolism was becoming a useful communication aid for him.

Details of the assessment and development of his language are as follows.

First assessment, aged 2 years

Receptive communication

There was no verbal comprehension at all. In fact he showed no awareness of a voice even when his mother spoke close to his ear. He did not watch faces for communication, but showed some recognition of facial expression. Communications had to be very direct and perceptually obvious for him to understand. He could follow some simple gross gesture, such as pointing, but no 'signs'.

Expressive communication

His vocalizations were simply expressions of emotion, with no attempt at any directed message. They consisted of vowel sounds, throaty sounds, and repetitive strings of 'a-wow-wow-wow'. They were often very loud, and not used for communication. He communicated either directly, or with gross gesture, and with a variety of facial expression.

Symbolic understanding

He did not use the representational toys at all for play, or as a language substitute. The doll-play material did not seem to be meaningful to him. The nearest he came to any sort of symbolism was in the use of gross gesture for communication, but this did not really even amount to mime.

Second assessment, aged 2.7 years

Receptive communication

He was a very socially aware and communicative child by this time, with no shyness. All communications still had to be very direct, or very obvious gestures accompanied by much facial expression. There was still no attempt at verbal comprehension and he did not look for this. During the tests he looked constantly for right–wrong cues in the form of head shakes and nods from the examiner, often deliberately doing something wrong as though to test this out. He sought his own feedback in this way by doing something wrong, shaking his head, then doing it right and clapping his hands. At this stage he was very dependent on this simple right–wrong feedback in all his understanding.

Expressive communication

He again made a great deal of noise in the form of squeals and grunts, but did not attempt any vocal communication. This was still mainly facial expression and gross gesture.

He was reported to have learnt one or two words which he produced silently using lips and tongue but no voice. These were 'Daddy' and 'thank you', but they could not be elicited during the session.

Symbolic understanding

This was still poorly developed for a 2½ year old child of average intelligence. He was just beginning to recognize some of the toys but did not attempt any sequential play, and some of his actions with the toys were bizarre. With the large doll-play material he brushed and combed the doll's hair, but put the cup and saucer on its head. With the small doll-play material he put the blanket on the bed, but did not use the doll; he turned the toy table upside down and put the chair on it.

Third assessment, aged 4.4 years

Receptive communication

By this time Mark had begun to achieve some verbal language and a more extensive understanding of gesture. With the aid of lip-reading he was able to select familiar objects and simple representational toys in response to naming. He was just beginning to be able to relate two named objects, (such as 'put the doll on the chair') but usually only managed to select one of the objects. The move from single verbal labels to relating two named objects is a big step for hearing-impaired children. They tend to assimilate the first operative word and then look away from the speaker to find the named object or toy. It needs a good deal of training to get them to keep looking at the speaker's face until the sentence is complete. Mark's verbal understanding did not go beyond the 'noun' stage, and he was not able to select objects by use.

Expressive communication

He was communicating by means of a combination of single words and symbolic gesture. There were occasional word-combinations such as 'where man?'. In terms of developmental age, his expressive vocabulary (2.8 year level) was well ahead of his ability for sentence construction (2.0 year level), which is a typical pattern for deaf children.

Symbolic understanding

He had by this time achieved a good understanding of symbols, and was using symbolic gesture freely to back up and extend his communications.

Fourth assessment, aged 5.9 years

Receptive communication

Since the age of 4.4 years he has made the equivalent of 7 months progress in verbal comprehension. This may seem a small improvement in 17 months, but it is approximately average progress for a child with this degree of hearing impairment. The move from following single words to following sentences containing more than one operative word, perhaps including verbs and other parts of speech, is very difficult for severely deaf children, and developmental progress is laboriously slow when they have to depend mainly on lip-reading. Mark used a combination of lip-reading and powerful hearing aids. He could now follow sentences including noun–verb combinations, and a few adjectives such as those referring to size and colour. He still failed with directions including more than two operative words. He is now beginning to read a little, which should considerably enhance his ability to understand sentences and build up his central language ability. For those deaf children who are intellectually able, an early introduction to reading is clearly an enormous advantage.

Expressive communication

He is now using short sentences, with a range of language extending beyond simple noun–verb combinations. His spoken vocabulary (age equivalent 3.2 years) is again well ahead of his ability for sentence construction (age equivalent 2.6 years).

Summary of progress

In Figure 6 (a graph of Mark's progress), certain developmental patterns typical of severely deaf children can be seen. First, there is no verbal language at all at 2 and $2\frac{1}{2}$ years; second, when verbal language begins, expressive language is consistently ahead of verbal comprehension; third, his expressive vocabulary is consistently ahead of his ability for sentence construction. What is not typical of deaf children was his slowness in developing symbolic understanding. Deaf children often develop early symbolic play, and use this as a language substitute, moving on to a spontaneous use of mime and gesture. When Mark did develop symbolic understanding he used this well with gesture, but he missed some of the early prelanguage experience of acting out sequences with symbolic toys.

In a study of 78 hearing-impaired children attending an assessment centre, the following findings are important.

(1) There was a tendency throughout the sample for expressive language to precede verbal comprehension in

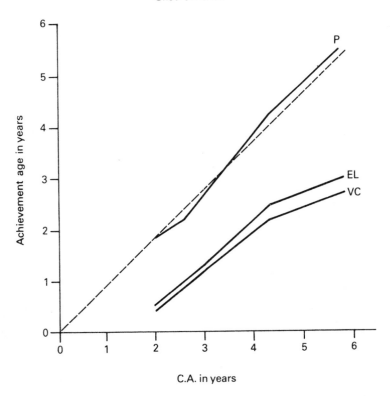

Figure 6   The dotted line shows the rate of non-verbal intellectual development at the first assessment. This was well maintained during the time he was followed up, as shown by the solid line P. The solid lines showing language progress illustrate the difficulty, for a severely deaf child, in moving beyond the early stages of verbal language development to a level greater than 3 years. Between 2 and 3 years the complexity of language increases considerably in normal development and these stages are particularly difficult for a deaf child. P: non-verbal performance abilities; E L: expressive language; VC: Verbal comprehension

terms of developmental age. This is understandable, because in the early stages of expressive language a child can use his limited store of central language in a variety of situations to communicate and express his ideas, but in following directions from others he must adapt to the language used by the speaker which may contain many words he has not learnt. An example is Tom, an intelligent, totally deaf 9 year-old, with excellent reading ability. He was asked (in writing) 'show me how the man walks into the field'. He made the man crash into the fence, using his own interpretation of the words 'walk into'. Without hearing, there is not the same opportunity for learning the variety of meaning that words can have.

(2) In expressive language, vocabulary developed well in advance of sentence construction. In severely deaf children, language learning is a completely different process from first-language learning in hearing children. It is learnt in many ways like a second language, when the concepts and symbolic understanding on which it depends have far outstripped the language that should go with them. With much labour, a verbal label is attached to a long-established concept such as 'big', instead of developing alongside the concept with mutual enhancement of both concept formation and language. So it is not surprising that verbal labels are learnt well in advance of other aspects of language, as they so often are in second-language learning.

(3) No child with severe hearing loss (greater than 70 db) achieved a verbal comprehension age greater than 3 years, and only two such children achieved an expressive language age greater than 3 years, during the time they were followed up (until 5 or 6 years).

(4) By a mental age of 3 to 4 years, none of these children had adequate verbal language to internalize as a useful thought process. This sets certain limits on the

development of some intellectual processes unless they are able to substitute some other form of symbolism. Most of the intelligent children used some form of symbols, either visual imagery, gestures, or a fully established sign system. One child with no language at the age of 7 years used to draw diagrams in the air to try to express his ideas both in communication and in thinking out practical tasks. Another child, aged 9 years, who had been taught the Paget–Gorman sign system, was attempting to match abstract animal forms. When she came to the crocodile, she signed 'animal' and then 'staircase', so forming a concept which enabled her to match animals with stair-like backs. These alternative strategies are intellectually important to children who cannot develop verbal language by the age when it usually becomes internalized as an intellectual process. This is now becoming increasingly recognized in teaching severely deaf children, but there are still some teachers who do not believe in the use of alternative systems.

A BLIND CHILD: DAVID

David has retrolental fibroplasia and is totally blind. He has no other handicaps except for a mild intellectual retardation. He was assessed at the age of 4.4 years on admission to a nursery school for blind children, and followed up for the next two years. At the time of admission there were behaviour problems at home, where he was reported to be destructive and wilful. At the first assessment the picture was not promising from the intellectual point of view, but with special help at the nursery school he made good progress, and by the age of 6 years he was already learning braille and was able to transfer to one of the schools for blind children, although still as a slow learner.

Language development and assessment

First assessment, aged 4.4 years

Behaviour

He was clearly very disturbed by the unfamiliar surroundings despite the presence of his parents. He was not able to settle to anything, but wandered restlessly about the room, feeling everything, but with no real interest in anything. He talked all the time to himself, using self-directive 'situational' phrases. Assessment was mainly by structured observation, as any attempt to get him to sit down and do anything specific caused great distress and anxiety.

Understanding of objects (performance)

He was interested in the screw-toys and enjoyed taking things apart, but he did nothing constructive. His play was explorative but mainly from a destructive point of view. Once he had taken something to pieces he lost interest in it.

Verbal comprehension

He was able to demonstrate a good deal of situational understanding, but he could not select any object in response to naming. He had clearly not reached the stage of understanding object labels, which is a considerable milestone for a blind child. He did not listen readily to speech. This aspect of his development was more retarded than any other area at that time, with an age equivalent, for a blind child, of 22 months.

Expressive language

He was able to name two of the test objects, but only after

a long delay. Naming objects is easier for a blind child than the receptive equivalent of selection in response to naming. Expressively, David was just beginning to achieve verbal labels. His spontaneous 'talk' consisted almost entirely of repetitive, emotive phrases reflecting adult control of his own behaviour, such as 'Don't break it, musn't pull apart'; 'hold it nicelip'; don't be naughty'; 'dass a hot fire'. Apart from a tenuous emotional relationship, these phrases had no connection with any action he was carrying out.

In general, he presented as a retarded blind child with an overall intellectual level of not more than $2\frac{3}{4}$ years for a blind child, and with a more marked specific retardation in verbal comprehension combined with a listening difficulty. A programme of early education was carried out to help his general progress and his specific difficulties, concentrating to a large extent on listening and attention, and on moving from destructive to constructive activities.

Second assessment, aged 5.4 years

After a year of intensive help at the nursery school for blind children, David had made some very encouraging progress (see Figure 7), with accelerated development in the important intellectual areas of verbal comprehension and constructional abilities. He was still doing a good deal of 'random' talking, but there was more meaningful expressive language than last time.

Behaviour

He was more settled generally, and no longer showed panic in unfamiliar situations. He was able to attend reasonably well to a learning task provided he had the one-to-one attention of an adult. His attention control was much better than a year ago, but still immature for his age.

Language development and assessment

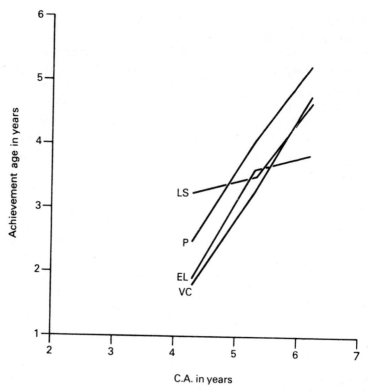

Figure 7   The graph shows the relatively high level of superficial language structure at the initial assessment as compared to the meaningful use of language and verbal comprehension. LS: language structure; P: non-verbal performance abilities; EL: meaningful use of expressive language; VC: verbal comprehension

Performance abilities

He was becoming more constructive with simple concrete material, and was beginning to match sizes and shapes, demonstrating the beginnings of understanding of abstract concepts.

Case studies

Verbal comprehension

This proved to be one of the most encouraging aspects of his development over the year. He was now able to listen reasonably well, provided an adult helped to control his attention, and to follow simple verbal directions. In the test situation he could select named objects, relate two named objects, and select some of the objects by use. His level was now 3.7 years by the standards for blind children.

Expressive language

Meaningful language was by now beginning to take over from his previous repetitive 'talk'. He still needed to repeat directions aloud sometimes, to help him assimilate and remember what was said to him. He was still using some pronoun reversals and was confused with some prepositions, but he could tell the use of objects on request, and make an attempt to construct a sentence about an ongoing activity.

Third assessment, aged 6.2 years

David had continued to make good progress, with some steady catching up towards his age level in most of the intellectual and language areas. His attention focus still needed firm adult control, but was steadily improving.

Concept formation

By now he had a good understanding of abstractions such as size, shape and position, and was able to sort 'same' and 'different'. This is a very adequate basis on which to build language.

Verbal comprehension

He was able to relate three named objects, to select objects by use, and was beginning to follow directions containing abstractions such as relative size, length, negatives and passive tenses. He had now achieved a level of 4.9 years in this aspect of language, by the standards for blind children.

Expressive language

He was able to construct good sentences without the need for repeating adult phrases, but there was still some immaturity in language use when he was requested to tell about an ongoing activity. He was also making good use of language in guiding his activities, which helped his thinking and attention.

Summary of progress

David's progress demonstrates many of the specific problems encountered by blind children in learning language. There is a particular difficulty with the stage of object labels. This stage is usually delayed, as compared to sighted children, with an enormous build-up of situational phrases before it is eventually reached. This occurs in receptive and expressive aspects of language. The reason for this is clear. Sighted children are constantly hearing the names of objects and people in the visual presence of those objects, so they have every chance of associating the word with its referant. This association does not happen with blind children unless a very insightful parent or teacher makes sure that the child actually handles the object on all the occasions it would normally be seen, and that it is clearly labelled for him at the same time. This exercise should be carried out in daily living activities whenever the object is used. For example, when it is time to brush the child's hair, he should be encouraged to handle the brush first, the adult saying 'here's your brush', 'let's brush your hair', at the same time helping the child to brush his own hair rather than taking the brush from him while the adult does the brushing. In this way he will be helped to learn object recognition, use of common objects, object labels, and telling the use of objects.

Blind children with fluent 'speech', such as David, often use this as a contact-keeping tool where a sighted child would use vision. It is a common experience when going into a nursery class for blind children for one or more of the children to approach the newcomer and say 'what's your name? . . .', 'Where do you live? . . .', 'Did you come in a car? . . .', 'What have you come for?'. These questions are repeated over and over again until the child has 'summed up' the newcomer in a way that a sighted child would do by staring at him for some time and looking him up and down. This 'scanning' use of speech often leads to apparently meaningless repetition of the same questions and phrases, and serves a different purpose from the truly linguistic use of speech. The two aspects of language, (a) language structure, and (b) vocabulary and content, are best assessed separately in blind children, because they may be at quite different developmental levels, as they were at the first assessment of David (see Figure 7).

It is very important that blind children should have help as early as possible in developing meaningful, object-related language, as this has to take over so many of the coordinating functions of vision.

A MENTALLY HANDICAPPED CHILD: RUTH

The range and degree of language handicaps among mentally handicapped children can vary just as much as in mentally normal children, and the types of language handicap are much the same. There is nothing specific or typical about early language development in mentally handicapped children as there is with blind or deaf children. Everything is delayed, as language is paced by intellectual development, so each stage of prelanguage and early language is more prolonged. As a case study Ruth, a young mongol child still at the prelanguage stages of development, was chosen. Many young mentally handicapped children need help in these early stages, to form a sound basis for the later development of language. They are often expected to 'talk' before they have this solid foundation of symbolic understanding and concept formation, with the result that, if they speak at all, their language expression remains superficial and repetitive in type. Research has shown that much can be done in the early stages to help these children, and Ruth is an example of this.

First assessment, aged 2.1 years

Ruth was an undersized mongol child who also had a cardiac murmur, a marked squint, and hypotonia, but her hearing and vision were considered to be adequate for early learning. At assessment, she presented as a friendly, happy little girl. Specific developmental areas were assessed as follows.

Attention control

She was still at the stage of fleeting attention, easily distracted by whatever caught her interest at the moment, and nothing held her attention for long. This is the earliest level of attention, typical of the first year of life.

Performance abilities

She was able to relate two objects, or two components, but not three. She could take objects out of containers, and put them in again with some encouragement, if the container was large enough (a shoe box, for instance), but she tended to throw things if left to herself. She needed training at this stage of putting two things together–such as lids onto boxes.

Symbolic understanding

She was able to demonstrate object recognition with real objects of the right size, and was just beginning to understand some of the large doll-play material.

Verbal comprehension

She could follow familar phrase patterns when all the usual clues were present, and would occasionally hand a named object on request, but her understanding of object labels was very unreliable.

Expressive language

She was a very vocal child who used plenty of jargon patterns, some of which were recognizable as situationally appropriate, for example, 'ee-ar'.

Ruth was admitted to a language clinic programme, making the parents the 'teachers', and incorporating early education into daily living activities at home (see Chapter 10). The speech therapist saw parents and child once every six weeks to give the parents further guidance. In this case, the aim was to help total intellectual development, including prelanguage, as Ruth did not have a specific language deficit as compared to her overall level.

The advice was related to the findings from the assessment, with work concentrated on understanding concrete material, forming a basis of early concepts including object recognition, and building up plenty of situational understanding at a prelanguage level. The specific recommendations are summarized below.

(1) Teach with only two objects or components at a time, such as objects in container, or container and lid. Check the throwing habit, and teach her instead to put things deliberately into containers.

(2) Consolidate the appropriate use of meaningful everyday objects, and move on to large doll-play, using the doll at appropriate times in the day, such as bathing the doll at Ruth's own bathtime, and feeding it at mealtimes.

(3) Consolidate her understanding of phrase patterns by deliberately linking specific phrases to specific situations, and rewarding an appropriate response. Lead her gradually on to an understanding of object labels.

(4) No need to work specifically on expressive language at this stage.

Second assessment, aged 3.1 years

Reference to the progress graph (Figure 8) will illustrate the very rapid progress that Ruth made over the year, with accelerated development in all areas of intellectual function and in language. There was also a very striking improvement in her ability for attention control, which proved to be a considerable learning asset. Progress in specific areas was reported as follows.

Attention control

Rapid improvement was made here, the equivalent of nearly 2 years' progress in this area. She now attended to adult directions and, with help, related them to what she was doing. She was able to sit and cooperate for quite a long time. Her interest was well held throughout the session, and she was able to adapt her attention focus from one test to another.

Performance abilities

She could now manage simple form boards, and put together a three-component model such as a box, lid and cubes. She demonstrated a learning readiness for the stage of two-category sorting.

Symbolic understanding

She was able to play well and meaningfully with the small doll-play material, and could match toys and pictures.

Verbal comprehension

She was by now reliable at selecting objects and toys in response to naming, and was beginning to be able to relate two named objects.

Expressive language

Her language expression was confined to single words or word combinations, but she used these appropriately, and was able to name some of the objects and pictures on request.

There will, of course, be certain limits set to the ultimate progress each mentally handicapped child can make, but this sort of early help can enable each child to make the best of such developmental potential he has, by making daily living activities appropriate learning experiences for each child.

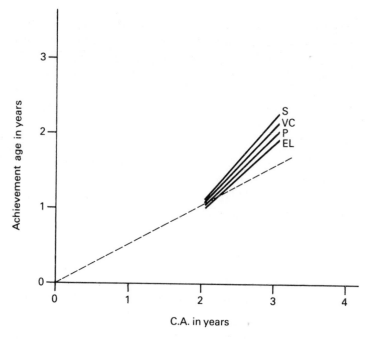

Figure 8   Ruth. The dotted line shows the progress rate on the basis of the first assessment. The solid lines show the progress rate during the year in which she attended the language clinic. Accelerated progress can be seen in the four developmental areas (1) non-verbal performance; (2) symbolic understanding; (3) verbal comprehension; and (4) expressive language. In all areas she made nearly a year's developmental progress in a year, which is very rapid progress for a child whose ability levels were initially only half her age. S: symbolic understanding; VC: verbal comprehension; P: non-verbal performance abilities; EL: expressive language

A CHILD WITH CEREBRAL PALSY: KAREN

Karen is very severely handicapped with cerebral palsy, affecting all four limbs and the control of her speech musculature. She has no controlled hand or arm movements and no possibility of developing coherent speech. She is, however, of near average intelligence, and able to make good use of eye-pointing and indications of 'yes' and 'no' for purposes of communication. Her vision and hearing are unimpaired, so she has plenty of opportunity to receive communications in the normal way. She was followed at intervals from the age of $7\frac{1}{2}$ months, and her parents had plenty of advice and help from a unit specializing in children with cerebral palsy.

First assessment, aged $7\frac{1}{2}$ months

Behaviour

She was very aware of strangers, and responded at first by a greatly increased stiffness of her arms and hands. At this stage she was able to use her right hand for reaching out for objects and holding them, but she seemed unaware of her left hand, and let fall any object put into it.

Performance abilities

She reached out for a red ring and a spoon, attempting to bring them to her mouth, demonstrating the establishment of sensory coordination at a 6 month level. Her head control was so poor that she had to be carefully positioned in order to scan objects on the table.

Response to sound

At this stage she was over-responsive to sound, so that care had to be taken not to make her jump. She turned her head to the source of sounds but could not always locate them directly. Her response to sound was selective in that she demonstrated a more positive (smiling) response to her mother's voice than to other sounds. This aspect of her intelligence was to develop into one of her most useful learning channels, and the one least interfered with by her extensive physical handicaps.

Vocalization

She was only able to produce vowel sounds, and did a great deal of abortive mouth opening.

Second assessment, aged 21 months

Progress was rather slow in these early months, despite the promise of low average intelligence at the previous assessment. This is not unusual with physically handicapped children in these early learning stages, when so much depends on learning through manipulation. Her hand use continued to be very limited. She was attempting a little bit of manipulation but it was such an effort for her that she often preferred just to watch. All tests had to be carried out using an eye-pointing response, even the performance tests, where she directed operations with her eyes.

Understanding of concrete objects

She was able to learn a simple one-to-one match, such as putting the round inset into the appropriate hole in a form board, and could relate one object to another by putting things into containers. All this was done by guiding the examiner's hands with her eye-pointing. She still did not manage to relate three things, such as box, lid and cube. She demonstrated a level of understanding equivalent to about two-thirds of her age.

Case studies

Verbal comprehension

She was able to recognize familiar situational phrases and, within the limits of her handicaps, to respond appropriately. She could also understand an occasional object label, again demonstrated by eye-pointing, selecting a brush, cup and spoon in response to naming. Her developmental level for this aspect of language was also about two-thirds of her age.

Third assessment, aged 3.6 years

By this age a more extensive assessment was possible. Although the physical limitations were just as great, she had learnt good communication with more reliable eye-pointing and an indication of 'yes' and 'no'. She still had no useful function in her hands and could not make any coherent speech sounds. Her level of understanding was scattered around three-quarters of her age, but varied greatly with different areas of learning. Her learning, and opportunities for intellectual development had, of course, been very patchy as a result of her extensive handicaps, despite the excellent help she had received from her parents and from the staff at the cerebral palsy unit. Details of her abilities and achievements at that time are as follows.

Performance understanding

She could manage a reversed three-hole form board, demonstrating a well-established matching ability for simple shapes. She could put together the three sets of box, lid and cubes from the Griffiths Scale, including matching the colours. This demonstrated good understanding of three-component models combined with colour matching. She could not put together a nest of cubes or build a tower with bricks in size order. This demonstrated a relatively immature understanding of size concept.

Use of abstractions for concept formation

In a task of matching abstract animal forms, which required bringing together and relating the three abstractions of size, shape and colour, she was able to achieve a level consistent with her age. She also managed to construct a wooden manikin from the separate pieces, putting the head, arms and legs in the right places. In this type of task, her relatively good intelligence was able to transcend the physical limitations, with an understanding that went beyond the directly perceptual.

Verbal comprehension

Using the Reynell Developmental Language Scales, Version B, a specifically adapted standardized scale for use with eye-pointing, Karen achieved a $2\frac{3}{4}$ year level, demonstrating that this is again a useful learning asset for her although still a little below average for her age.

She went on to attend a school for physically handicapped children where she continued to make good progress, using a specially adapted typewriter for communication.

Summary of progress

Karen's case illustrates how important it is to establish and develop all possible communication systems with children who have such extensive handicaps, blocking the usual forms of language development. It also shows how important it is to establish the true language ability from the point of view of receptive and internalized language, despite the expressive limitations. It would have been

very easy to underestimate Karen by a too supe_
examination.

Karen's central language and verbal comprehension were relatively good, with the limitations mainly due to poor muscular control in the expressive aspects. It must be understood, however, that children with cerebral palsy in general are at risk for all types of language handicap, including 'central' language problems, as there is cerebral involvement. It is particularly important, therefore, to sort out exactly what the extent of the language and communication problem is, what the developmental possibilities are, and to arrange for appropriate help as soon as possible.

A CHILD WITH DEVELOPMENTAL LANGUAGE HANDICAP: JAMES

James was referred at the age of $3\frac{1}{2}$ years for delayed language development. There were no other handicaps apart from some immaturity in manipulative and motor skills. There was nothing in the developmental history or the environment to account for the language delay, so it was considered to be a specific developmental delay. The psychological assessment indicated average intelligence for non-verbal performance abilities, but with a marked delay in both aspects of language development (receptive and expressive), and problems with attention control. He presented, in fact, with a typical pattern of an early developmental language handicap.

First assessment, aged $3\frac{1}{2}$ years

James was a friendly and responsive little boy, making good use of such communication abilities as he had. A breakdown of his abilities at that time is as follows.

Attention control

This was one of his greatest learning difficulties. He seemed to slip easily in and out of attention 'focus'. When his attention was focused on what he was doing he could manage a reasonable level of function, but he tended to lose his attention and start responding at random. At these times it was often difficult to get his attention back. Developmentally his attention was at a level more usually encountered in the second year of life, so was an area of considerably immaturity for him, needing a great deal of help.

Non-verbal performance abilities

He was able to achieve his best level with concrete material, where the material itself helped to hold his attention, and where he did not need to be confused by verbal directions. Even with this type of material, however, he tended to forget what he was supposed to be doing and go off onto his own building.

Symbolic understanding and concept formation

He was able to make good use of imaginative play material, and to match toys and pictures, indicating a reasonably stable prelanguage basis, but he had difficulty with any intellectual task extending beyond what was explicit from the concrete material itself. There seemed to be no internalized symbolic process yet to help him with this.

Verbal comprehension

He carried on his own play with the test material, and had very great difficulty in integrating verbal directions. He often repeated the directions without understanding them. He was fairly reliable at selecting objects in response to naming, but could not manage anything more difficult. Typical of his difficulty in integration was his response to the request to 'put the car in the box'. He repeated 'car . . . box', but failed to relate this to the material.

Expressive language

His speech was inclined to be imitative, with a good deal of jargon, but there were some recognizable phrase patterns which were situationally appropriate. He had no difficulty in producing speech sounds, but they were often wrongly coded in words. For example: sots = sock, buch = brush, widow = window.

Intellectual use of language

He 'talked' as he played, but this was mainly repetitive phrases or jargon patterns. He could not use his own or adult verbalization as a directive to integrate his practical activities.

James, at that time, had a serious language handicap which needed immediate and intensive help if he was to have any chance of overcoming the difficulty by school age. He was admitted to a preschool language class which he attended for two hours daily throughout school terms.

Second assessment, aged 4½ years

James had a very successful year in the language class. He adapted quickly and soon became an integrated member of the group. He enjoyed the company of the other children and played well with them. The second assessment was carried out at the end of a year in the class. He showed very striking progress all round (Figure 9). All his

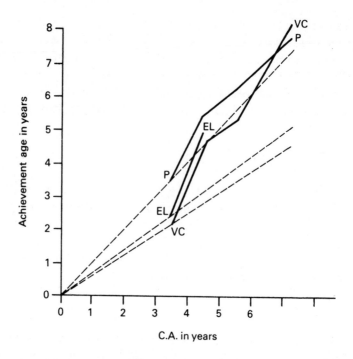

Figure 9   James. The dotted lines show the progress rate on the basis of the first assessment at the age of 3½ years. The solid lines show the actual rate of progress on the basis of follow-up assessments. The greatly accelerated progress after admission to the language class can be seen in both aspects of language development. This improved rate of progress was maintained after transfer to ordinary school at the age of 5 years. P: non-verbal performance abilities; VC: verbal comprehension; EL: expressive language

abilities, both intellectual and language, were by this time ahead of his age, and his attention control was no longer immature for his age. A breakdown of his abilities was as follows.

Attention control

He had achieved a level consistent with his age. He was able to sustain well-integrated attention for short spells, controlling his own attention focus, and assimilating directions while carrying out a task.

Non-verbal performance abilities

He achieved a level well above the average for his age, carrying out the tasks with good application of attention.

Concept formation

He had now learnt to use internalized concepts in thinking rather than depending only on perceptual matching.

Verbal comprehension

He could now reach a level of understanding well up to his age. He was able to follow verbal directions containing up to three 'operative' words, including the understanding of different parts of speech such as adjectives and prepositions, but there was still some confusion with longer directions.

Expressive language

He talked all the time, and was now fluent in expressing his ideas although there were still some immaturities in sentence construction. He was able to verbalize plenty of ideas when talking about pictures, as shown in the following example: 'He's havin a puddin . . . he's goin to eat it up'.

Intellectual use of language

He had moved rapidly through the stage of talking aloud in directing and integrating his own activities, and had been able to internalize this intellectual use of a language so that it was now a useful vehicle for thought.

Following this assessment a recommendation was made for a transfer to ordinary school at the end of term.

Third assessment, aged 5½ years

He had settled well at school, and his abilities at assessment were summarized as follows.

His test responses showed that there were still traces of his languages difficulty when the demands were at a high level. His father reported that he still could not verbalize his thoughts as quickly as he was able to think, when trying to tell about an event. He achieved an above-average level on performance tests, and an average level on tests of verbal intelligence. This balance was reversed later on, as the findings of the fourth assessment showed (see below).

Fourth assessment, aged 7¼ years

By this time James had overcome all his previous language difficulties and was proving himself to be a very 'verbal' child. His verbal intelligence was slightly above his performance intelligence, and he was reading at a level beyond his age. The scores were recorded as follows:

Verbal IQ 116
Performance IQ 111
Graded word reading test 7.9 years
Reading comprehension 9.5 years

James showed a typical pattern of a child with a developmental language delay without other handicaps, both in the pattern of his abilities at the first assessment and in his progress in response to early help.

In the early stages there are difficulties with receptive and expressive language, and with attention control. Attention control and verbal comprehension usually recover first, with expressive language taking a little longer. In James's case, the improvement was so rapid that both aspects of language were up to his age by the second assessment, as was his attention control, so the usual intermediate stage was no longer evident. The detailed records kept by the class teacher, however, showed that verbal comprehension was consistently ahead of expressive language until expressive language caught up towards the end of the year. James still showed some persisting difficulties at the age of 5½ years, but only when the higher levels of language use were required of him, and this did not interfere with his school work. These small remaining difficulties had completely cleared up at the final assessment, when he showed himself to be a really 'verbal' child with well-integrated verbal thinking and good verbal expression.

Summary of progress

The importance of early intervention for children with this type of handicap has been shown by the findings of the research study quoted in Chapter 10. The proportion of the 'no help' group who made a spontaneous recovery was strikingly smaller than the proportion of the experimental group who achieved this rapid progress. James's early language and attention difficulties were affecting whole areas of his intellectual make-up, and initially it was only in dealing with simple concrete material that he was able to achieve a level consistent with his age. After a year of intensive help, focused mainly on attention and verbal comprehension, he had made accelerated progress all round, and resolved his language difficulties to the extent that his language levels were consistent with his age. Perhaps most important of all, he had completely over-come his early severe attention problems which were affecting all aspects of learning.

James was selected for illustration of a developmental language handicap because he showed so many of the typical features. It should be understood, however, that there are many variations in early language handicaps, as indicated in Chapter 4, and they do not all follow the same pattern. The most obvious difficulties are usually in expressive language, and this is often the reason for referral. Among such children referred to an assessment centre it was found that the problem was confined to expressive language in only 25 per cent of the children with a so-called 'specific' language handicap. The large majority had problems also in verbal comprehension and in other language-related areas such as attention control. A comprehensive assessment is essential in order to define the developmental areas in need of help.

PLOTTING PROGRESS

In all the cases quoted in this chapter, the progress graphs (Figures 6, 7, 8 and 9) are based on the findings from standardized tests, so it is possible to plot age equivalents for different areas of development. Many clinicians will not have access to these specialized assessment tools, but progress can still be assessed in this way by referring to the stages of development described in Chapters 5 and 6, and the approximate ages given for each. In this way it will be possible to see whether the child is making satisfactory progress at each of the follow-up assessments.

Case studies

The developmental assessment tools used in the case studies are:

(1) Verbal comprehension and expressive language: Reynell Developmental Language Scales (Reynell, 1977)
(2) Non-verbal performance abilities: Griffiths Scale (Griffiths, 1970)
(3) Concept formation, symbolic understanding and attention control: as described by the author in other publications (Cooper, Moodley and Reynell, 1978)
(4) Assessment of visually handicapped children: Reynell–Zinkin Scales (Reynell, 1979)

Chapter 10

REMEDIAL MEASURES

It seems fitting to devote this last chapter to a short description of a study which was carried out at The Wolfson Centre on intervention procedures for young children with early language handicaps, and to the findings from this study. The whole purpose of understanding and assessing early language development, from the point of view of the clinician, must surely be to provide some effective means of helping the children. The findings from this study show that early help for language-handicapped children is very effective in accelerating their rate of language development to the extent that the large majority can take their place in ordinary school and make satisfactory progress there when the time comes. These findings enhance the importance of the role of the clinician in identifying the children who need help at an early age.

The study was carried out between 1973 and 1978, and has been fully described (Cooper et al., 1979), so only a summary of the points relevant to this book will be presented here.

The aim was to select children who showed evidence of a specific language delay, between the ages of 2 and 5 years, to give intensive help either via the parents under the direction of a speech therapist, or in a small language class under the direction of a teacher.

The philosophy upon which the Developmental Language Programme (DLP) was based can be summed up in the following quotation (Reynell, 1976):

Early education is part of, and integrated with total living. It is not confined to certain hours of the day, or days of the week, but depends on creating a total educational environment so that each child, whatever his handicaps, may be able to use each daily living experience to promote and enrich his development. It is the role of those who are professionally concerned with education and development to work with the parents so that this early education may take place in the most appropriate way.

THEORETICAL BASIS

The procedures were based on the model in Figure 10.

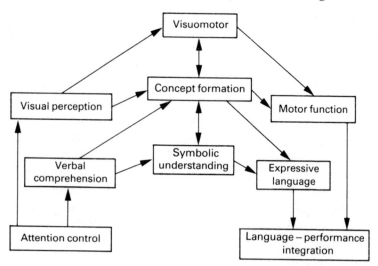

Figure 10   Model used as basis for language intervention programmes

Each of the developmental areas in this model are related to early language development, and the interrelation between these areas is shown. Each area is broken down into developmental stages covering the range $1\frac{1}{2}$ to 5 years, which are the important years for language development. The programme of help depends on consolidating learning and understanding at whatever stage the child has reached, in each area, and helping him on to the next stage of development, while at the same time maintaining an appropriate balance between the whole. For example, when teaching verbal comprehension, it is important to understand and use whatever level the child has reached in concept formation and symbolic understanding. It is useless to teach the words 'long' and 'short' unless the child has a real understanding of these concepts, and can sort long and short objects into two categories. It is also useless to use pictures for teaching language until the child has reached the stage of symbolic understanding when the pictures become meaningful.

It is not expected for the parents carrying out the programme to understand the theory, but it is necessary that whoever is directing and guiding the programme should do so. It is the role of the speech therapist or teacher to translate this into practical everyday activities. The parents can then be shown how to bring appropriate learning into everyday living. They are shown how to use whatever attention the child is able to give, what sort of material to use, and how to talk to him. Real life situations such as mealtimes are used. Learning at all stages can be built into these situations, and however busy a mother is she still has to feed, bath and bed her child. At the prelanguage stages the parents are helped to use patterned phrases for each regularly occurring event such as 'here's your mug, have a drink'. Early symbolic understanding can be helped by using a large doll or teddy, sitting it beside the child at mealtimes and 'feeding' it at the same time. Later, the child can learn to follow simple requests such as 'put the biscuit on the plate', 'give Daddy a cake'. The parents will be shown how to get the child's full attention before giving these verbal directions, to talk about here-and-now situations, and how to monitor their own speech so that the child is able to assimilate the directions.

The programme can equally well be carried out in a small class, using the same basic idea applied to ordinary nursery school activities. Plenty of play with small representational toys is appropriate as this lends itself well to all stages of language learning.

THE SETTING

Parent programme

Parent and child attended the clinic once every 6 weeks for a session with the speech therapist. Sometimes both parents attended, and sometimes another adult who had responsibility for the child's daily care. The sessions took the form of not only showing the parents how to use daily living experiences for language learning, but also getting them to carry this out under supervision. This led to much better understanding and carry-over than merely explaining what to do. Whenever possible real situations were used, such as dressing, or having an orange drink, and the scope was widened with the use of dolls when the child was ready for that sort of symbolic understanding. Each session lasted about an hour, which included taking the family down to the waiting room for coffee, putting on coats and toileting. This was considered to be all part of the practical situation which was used for creating an appropriate language learning environment.

Class programme

There were two classes, with eight children in each, under the direction of a teacher and nursery assistant. Each class met every day during school term, one class in the mornings and one in the afternoons; the session lasted 2 hours.

The children

The Wolfson Centre children had specific language handicaps such that their language age was not more than two-thirds of their non-verbal performance age. Severely deaf children and those with severe physical handicaps were excluded. The age range for the class children was 3 to $4\frac{1}{2}$ years on admission (50 children), and of the 'clinic' children 2 to $4\frac{1}{2}$ years (69 children).

The children in the Field Trial class studies (31 children) presented with a wide range of intellectual handicaps, and were older than the Wolfson Centre children, with an age range up to $10\frac{1}{2}$ years. The Field Trial 'clinic' children (27) were comparable in age and handicaps to the Wolfson Centre sample.

ASSESSMENTS

Ongoing records of progress

These were kept by the teacher or speech therapist, to make sure that the immediate aims were achieved for each child in each of 12 developmental areas related to language development. These record sheets were so designed that each developmental stage was set out for each of the 12 developmental areas so that whoever was directing the programme could see immediately what her aims were for each particular child and whether there was progress.

Quantitative annual assessments

These were carried out to assess the rate of progress in the five areas for which there are age-equivalent scores. These are attention control, symbolic understanding and concept formation, performance (non-verbal), verbal comprehension, and expressive language. Progress was rated as 'good' (accelerated), 'steady' (no change in rate), or 'poor' (decelerating) (Figure 11).

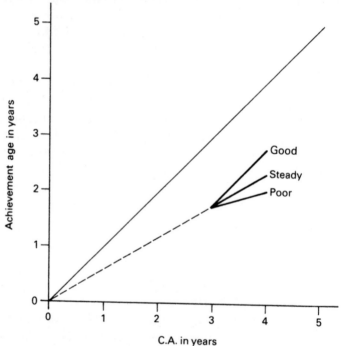

Figure 11   Examples of good, steady and poor progress between the ages 3 and 4 years

In order to separate the three groups quantitatively it was necessary to decide on a cut-off point. An arbitrary point was chosen such that 'steady' progress over a year included the equivalent of one year's progress for that child, plus or minus three months. Anything outside these limits was rated as 'good' or 'poor' (Figure 12).

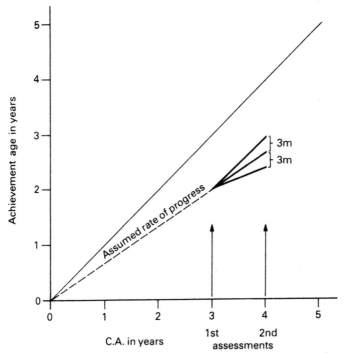

Figure 12   The range of 'steady' progress; assumed rate plus or minus 3 months over the year

The equivalent of a year's progress was estimated according to the assumed previous rate of development. For example, a 3-year-old child presenting with a language age of 2 years is assumed to have progressed at a rate of two-thirds his age in previous years. If this rate is increased, so that he makes two-thirds of a year plus 4 months or more during a year in treatment, this is rated as 'good' progress. In this way, the progress rate was assessed in the five measurable areas related to language development, and the children were divided into the three categories of 'good', 'steady' or 'poor' progress. These categories were used as a basis for validation. Anything less than 'good' progress in any aspect of development initially delayed was considered a failure from the point of view of the DLP.

RESULTS

Ongoing recordings

Summaries of the regular records made by the teacher on each child were related to the child's subsequent progress and adjustment after transfer to school, as reported by the receiving class teacher. Despite the initially severe language handicaps with which the children presented, and many associated handicaps of lesser degree, the teachers' reports indicated that 70 per cent of the whole class sample (50 children) made average to good progress in ordinary school during the first year after transfer.

For the purpose of validating the language class aims in terms of the 12 developmental areas worked on, the children were grouped according to programme achievement at the end of their time in the class, and these groups were related to subsequent teachers' reports on transfer to school. The groups were as follows:

Group A: School readiness achieved in all 12 areas. The eight children in this group were considered to be more than school ready on transfer at the age of five years, and were expected to do well at school.

Group B: School readiness achieved in 9 to 11 areas out of the 12. These 17 children were expected to adjust reasonably well to ordinary school and to make average progress.

Group C: School readiness achieved in five to eight of the 12 areas. Other areas still not school ready.

These children were expected to have some difficulties at first in ordinary school.

Group D: School readiness achieved in not more than four of the 12 areas. These children were expected to need special help or special schooling.

Table 5 shows that these groupings related closely to subsequent school adjustment and achievement.

Table 5 The relationship between school readiness groups and adjustment to school during the first term of transfer, as reported by the receiving teachers

School readiness group	Report of school adjustment				
	Good	Average	Difficult	Special school	Total
A	5	2	1	0	8
B	1	14	2	0	17
C	0	7	3	3	13
D	0	1	1	4	6
Total	6	24	7	7	44

N.B. Six children were not included in these figures because they were still under school age on leaving the class.

Conclusion: The individual aims and recording procedures are valid and realistic in relation to school progress and adjustment.

Measurement of rate of progress

Assessment of the rate of progress on each child, in the

five measurable areas, determined the success of the DLP in relation to individual children.

Language class sample: Progress in class

Figure 13 shows that the large majority of children made accelerated progress during their time in the language class in all five areas. The progress is less striking in non-verbal performance than in the other areas more closely related to language development. The reason for this is clear, as the children, by selection, were not

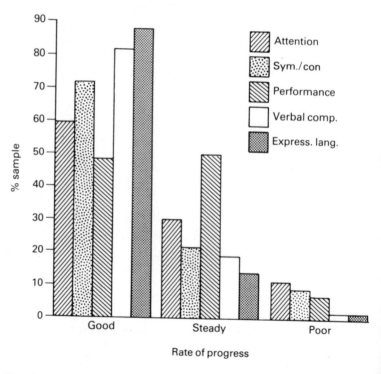

Figure 13   The rate of progress of the language class children during their time in the class, for the five measurable areas of development

specifically delayed in performance on entry, so there was less expectation of a change in the rate of this aspect of development. Work was focused on other areas which are more closely related to language development. In a way this acts as a 'control' to show the greater changing rate in the language-related areas.

Language class sample: Progress on follow up

Having shown that the children made accelerated progress during their time in the class, it was necessary to show that this improved rate of progress was maintained on follow up after leaving the class. As might be expected, there was some relative slowing down of the rate of progress on starting school, but a comparison of the overall rate of development from entry into the DLP to the final follow-up showed that the advantages gained in the class had been maintained; this is illustrated in Figure 14.

Language class sample: Areas specifically delayed

On admission to the DLP not all children showed a specific delay in all four language-related areas as compared to their non-verbal performance level. As the aim was to accelerate development particularly in the delayed areas, it is reasonable to expect the greatest progress in these aspects of development. Figure 15 shows the rate of progress of those children in the language class sample who initially showed specific delays.

The results are very striking. Nearly all the children showing initial specific delays accelerated their progress in those developmental areas, and this was maintained at the final assessment a year after leaving the class.

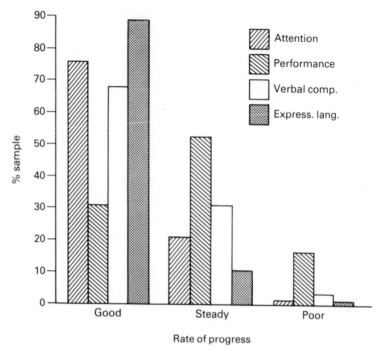

Figure 14 The rate of progress for the language class sample between the time of admission to the Developmental Language Programme, and the final follow-up after leaving the class

Language 'clinic' sample: Progress in clinic

Figure 16 and 17 show the progress of the 69 children in the language 'clinic' sample, first of all the whole sample, and then for those children who initially showed specific delays.

Again, the large majority of the children showed accelerated progress during treatment in all the language-related aspects of development.

Conclusion: The children in both the Wolfson Centre

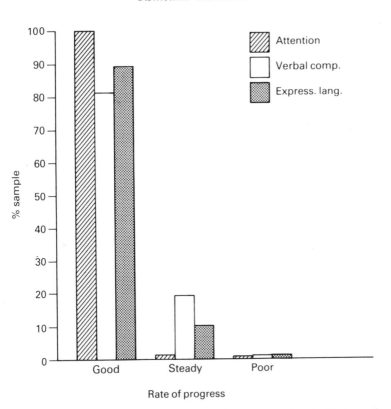

Figure 15 The rate of progress between the initial and final assessments for those children in the language class who initially showed specific delays

samples showed very striking acceleration in both aspects of language development and in the related areas of attention control and symbolic understanding. The procedures are therefore valid in relation to the aims for individual children.

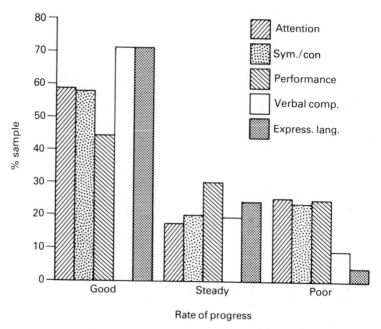

Figure 16 The rate of progress of the language 'clinic' children during their time in treatment

Group comparisons: Descriptions

In order to validate the DLP further, it was necessary to find out (a) whether it was effective in different settings outside the Wolfson Centre, and when carried out by different people, and (b) how the progress of the 'programme' children compared with those having no help, or having a more conventional type of speech therapy.

Field trials: language class

We were approached by teachers in some special classes and schools asking for help in setting up a language programme. These teachers agreed to carry out a field trial

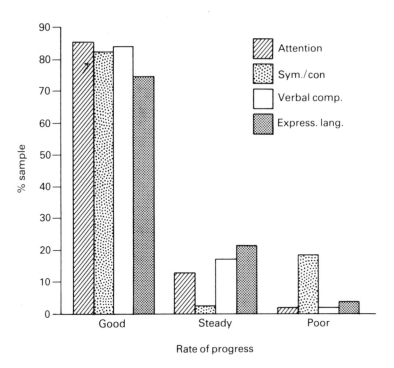

Figure 17   The rate of progress of those children in the language 'clinic' sample who initially showed specific delays

over a year. The before and after assessments were carried out by the Wolfson Centre team who also monitored the carrying out of the programme, but the actual work was done by the teachers in their normal local authority setting. The units included an ESN(S) school, an ESN(M) school, an assessment unit in ordinary school, and a preschool unit attached to a special school. There were a few 'dropouts' due to school transfer during the programme, but it was possible to follow 31 children in this sample. All had some degree of specific language handicap as compared to their non-verbal abilities, but not to the same degree as the Wolfson Centre children.

Field trials: Language 'clinic'

Local authority speech therapists in counties within reasonable reach of the London area were invited to take part. Twenty-seven children were selected for this field trial sample on the basis of age and handicap comparable to the Wolfson Centre children. Fifteen different speech therapists were involved. Progress was assessed over a year for all these field trial children.

Control groups

There were two control groups, (1) 20 children who were referred to the Wolfson Centre before any help was available, either at the centre or in their local authority. These children had a before and after assessment (one year between assessments) without any help for their language handicaps. They were equivalent in age and handicap to the Wolfson Centre experimental groups, so constituted an appropriate control. (2) The second group consisted of 39 children, also of equivalent age and handicap, who were having conventional weekly speech therapy in their local authority settings but were not 'programme' children. One-third of this sample consisted of Wolfson Centre referrals, and others were not. In every way, except for the programme followed, these children were comparable to the language 'clinic' field trial children.

Group comparisons: Results

Tables 6 and 7 show the percentage of each sample making accelerated progress in verbal comprehension and expressive language.

Conclusion: With the exception of the ESN(S) children who need longer than a year in treatment, the rate of

Table 6 The percentage of each sample making accelerated progress in the Wolfson Centre language class, and in the other, field classes, as compared to the children who had no help

Sample	Number of children	% accelerated progress	
		Verbal comprehension	Expressive language
Control group 1, no help	20	30	30
ESN(S) class	10	40	20
ESN(M) class	7	71	71
Assessment unit	8	88	63
TWC language class	50	82	86

Table 7 Comparing the percentage of each sample making accelerated language progress in the following groups: (a) control group 1, no help; (b) control group 2, conventional weekly speech therapy; (c) field trial language clinic sample and (d) Wolfson Centre language clinic sample

Sample	Number of children	% accelerated progress	
		Verbal comprehension	Expressive language
Control group 1, no help	20	30	30
Control group 2, conventional speech therapy	39	53	54
Field trial language clinic	27	60	70
TWC language clinic	69	72	72

progress in both aspects of language development in all groups using the DLP is better than either control group. The conclusion is that the procedures are valid in relation to the aims, and are adaptable to a number of different settings in both class and clinic.

RELATION TO DEGREE OF HANDICAP AND ASSOCIATED HANDICAPS

Accelerated progress occurred in children with all degrees of language handicap, and there was no evidence that it was related to the degree. There was also no clear relationship to the paediatric categories of 'causal' and 'developmental' (Sonksen, 1977). Children in both of these categories made accelerated progress. The only significant factor found was intellectual level. Children with a non-verbal performance IQ below 65 needed longer in treatment to achieve an equivalent proportion of accelerated language progress to the other children, but they did achieve this after 2 to 2½ years. Significant acceleration in attention control was achieved even in these retarded children during the first year.

Figure 18 shows that the children in the Wolfson Centre language class were only slightly below the normal population in non-verbal intelligence, whereas the language 'clinic' children were, as a group, considerably below this, with one-third of the sample having performance IQs below 65. This proved to be of significance in relation to the length of time needed to achieve accelerated language development.

Table 8 shows the percentage of each intellectual group making accelerated progress in one year, and in longer treatment. The figures show quite clearly that the children of lower intelligence take longer to achieve accelerated progress in some of the language-related aspects of development.

This is shown most clearly in Table 9. These figures are derived by subtracting the percentage making accelerated progress in the first year from the percentage making

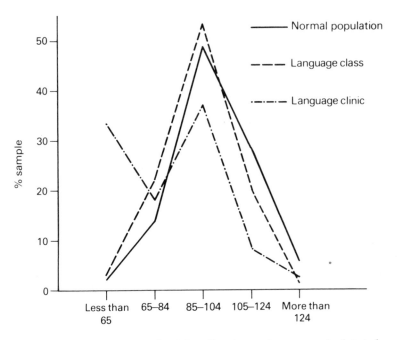

Figure 18   Showing the distribution of non-verbal intelligence in three groups of children

accelerated progress in longer treatment. Taking a 10 per
cent difference as an arbitrary point for 'significance', it
can be clearly seen that children with a performance IQ of
less than 65 make significantly better progress in both
aspects of language and in symbolic understanding when
in treatment for more than a year. Good progress in
attention control is achieved in one year even with this
group.

Children who are only moderately retarded (performance IQ 65 to 84) made good progress during the first
year in all aspects of language-related development, but
significantly more in expressive language after the first
year of treatment. Those of average intelligence or above,
showed rapid improvement in all aspects of language-

Table 8 The relation between performance IQ on admission to the language 'clinic' and rate of language progress. The figures show the percentage of each intellectual group making accelerated progress in 1 year and in more than 1 year of treatment, for the five measurable developmental areas

Performance IQ	First year only					More than 1 year				
	Att	S/C	P	VC	EL	Att	S/C	P	VC	EL
Less than 65	52	20	50	52	35	48	52	55	74	57
65 to 84	55	55	73	67	58	55	64	64	75	75
More than 84	66	58	25	68	74	69	60	34	71	82

Att Attention control
S/C Symbolic understanding and concept formation
P   Performance, non-verbal
VC   Verbal comprehension
EL   Expressive language

related development during the first year. This reflects the developmental pattern of recovery from a language handicap, with the prelanguage aspects of attention and symbolic understanding improving first, followed by verbal comprehension, and with expressive language recovering last.

These findings related to intellectual level explain the apparently disappointing progress of the children in the ESN(S) field trial group in the first year. Progress after a further year showed much better results (figures not shown here) in those children who had this opportunity. Conclusion: The DLP is appropriate for all types and degrees of early central language handicaps, but children who are severely intellectually retarded need more than a year in treatment.

Table 9 The difference in improvement rates between first year and full time. Figures represent the per cent accelerated progress in full time treatment minus the per cent accelerated progress in the first year. Figures in bold type indicate a difference in the improvement rate of more than 10 per cent for more than 1 year as compared to only 1 year

Performance IQ	Att	S/C	P	VC	EL
Less than 65	−4	**32**	5	**22**	**22**
65 to 84	0	9	−9	8	**11**
More than 84	3	2	9	3	8

DISCUSSION AND PRACTICAL IMPLICATIONS

The project set out to find and prove an effective way of helping language development in children with early language handicaps. The aim was to give the children as intensive help as possible during the early years by either (a) daily help in a language class, or (b) using the parents as teachers in daily living activities at home.

A developmentally rational programme was devised, so that the child's progress could be guided stage by stage in a number of areas of development closely related to language.

The procedures proved to be successful in accelerating language development in the class and in the parent (clinic) programme at the Wolfson Centre. They were then tried out in a number of different settings in the field trials, and proved to be successful and adaptable.

Validation studies strongly suggest that the developmental language programme is effective, and that the successes are due to the procedures as such, rather than to extraneous factors such as selection of children or professional personnel.

It is with some confidence, therefore, that these procedures are now published as a suggested guide to professional people who are concerned to help children with early language handicaps. The following discussion considers the use to be made of these findings.

Economic considerations

Special language classes are expensive, and may only be possible in large cities. However, the success rate among the class children was outstandingly high, so this is perhaps the most effective setting for early intervention with children who can manage a group situation. A 2-hour session 5 days a week proved as effective as a full 5-day week for young children. In our experience, regular daily attendance was much more effective than 1, 2 or 3 days a week. It is suggested, therefore, that if local facilities allow, a preschool class meeting for half a day 5 days a week, would be rewarding in terms of the language progress of the children, and may prevent continuing difficulties during the school years. With full time staff, it is suggested that there should be two classes, each of ten children, one meeting in the mornings and one in the afternoons.

Language classes in special schools would be another way of using resources and, in our experience, these were effective.

A third possibility is to use the DLP within the ordinary class setting in a special school, for those children who are language handicapped. This is now being tried in one of our field trial schools. In this case the language teacher plays a peripatetic role in guiding the class teachers throughout the school.

Although the success rate for the 'clinic' children in the

parent programme was less striking, it was still very high, and this is clearly the most economical way of using resources. Also, a wider range of young children can be helped, as it includes children from the age of 2 years, and children who for other reasons may not be able to manage a group situation.

In terms of speech therapists' time, the DLP allows many more children to have help, and to have it more intensively than the more conventional once-a-week therapy. Language education is incorporated into daily living activities by the parents, who are guided by a session with a speech therapist once every 6 weeks. Seeing three children a day in this 6-weekly programme enables each speech therapist to carry a case load of 90 children, giving constant help via the parents. This is more than twice the number that most speech therapists can manage on weekly therapy.

Apart from the simple economics, the success rate was higher for the children seen at 6-weekly intervals in the DLP than for those having conventional weekly speech therapy. This applied when the programme was carried out at the Wolfson Centre and when it was directed by a local speech therapist in a field trial situation.

The conclusion, in terms of the provision of facilities, is that the suggested programme should be viable under present circumstances without necessarily increasing the number of teachers or speech therapists, and that it should enable teachers and speech therapists to make appropriate and effective use of the time available in helping children with early language handicaps.

Type of child

The programme was designed for preschool children presenting with a specific language handicap, excluding the severely deaf, severely autistic and severely physically handicapped. Children with minor degrees of these handicaps were included, as was a wide range of intellectual handicap.

It was no surprise to find that ESN(S) children, both in the class situation and in the parent programme, needed a longer time for treatment to be effective than did those who were only mildly handicapped or who were of normal intelligence. In terms of intellectual progress, a year of remedial provision for an ESN(S) child may be equivalent to only one term for a child who is developing at a normal rate. We found that in 2 to 3 years these very retarded children made a language acceleration equivalent to that made by the intellectually normal children in 1 year. It can be concluded, therefore, that intellectual retardation is no reason for excluding the children from the DLP, provided that they are able to continue for 2 to 3 years.

Analysis of the reasons for 'failure', with the few children who did not make accelerated language progress, suggested that this was not due to the type of child, but rather to unusual social or emotional circumstances which prevented regular attendance or full cooperation.

Older children (7+ years), of normal or near normal intelligence, who have a very specific and persisting difficulty in language or articulation, need a different sort of approach and were not included in any of our samples. By the time they are intellectually about 7 years, all other cognitive processes have moved beyond the stages with which the DLP is concerned, and the children can usually manage a more direct focus on their particular difficulty in a one-to-one situation with a speech therapist. A few of the children in our sample needed this further help once their central language difficulties had resolved, usually to 'tidy up' remaining articulation problems.

Long-term effectiveness

Owing to limitations of staff and time available, it was only possible to follow up a small sample (38 children) after discharge, to see whether the language advantages were maintained. If the language level had reverted to that expected from the initial rate of development, clearly the intervention would have failed. The findings on this sample of children showed very strikingly that the advantages gained in the language class were maintained when reassessment was carried out from 6 to 30 months after discharge. There was some slowing down of the rate of development during the first year in school, which is to be expected, but a comparison of the rate of language progress at the final follow-up assessment with the initial rate of progress on entry into the programme, showed that the overall advantage had been maintained despite this temporary slowing down. The success rate in terms of maintained accelerated language progress was 80 to 90 per cent for the children in the sample who were initially significantly language delayed, and 100 per cent for resolution of problems of attention control.

The aim of the programme with preschool children was to improve the rate of language development, and to resolve the central language problems to the extent that language progress was firmly established and would continue. By the age of five years, children normally have this firm basis of language which becomes internalized as an intellectual process and so should not revert as do some more superficial skills when help is withdrawn. This proved to be the case with the sample of language handicapped children followed up. There is every reason to consider this sample representative of all the programme children, and a success rate of 80 to 90 per cent must surely be meaningful even in a small sample of 38 children.

These findings are reinforced in a more general way by the school adjustment and progress of the language class children after transfer; 70 per cent of the whole sample (50 children) were rated by their teachers as making good progress in ordinary school during the first year after transfer.

We may conclude that the developmental language programme is effective in accelerating language development, and in establishing a firm basis for further development in children who initially present with a significant language handicap.

CONCLUSION

There are many different types of language programme now, some of which are suitable for children in the early developmental stages with which this volume is concerned. The Developmental Language Programme described here is just one example, and has been quoted at some length because the validation studies seem to establish that efforts to help young children who have early language handicaps can be both effective and worthwhile. Every child in need should have this help, and it is often the responsibility of the local clinician to identify such children initially. It is hoped that this volume will help clinicians in this very important and responsible role.

APPENDIX I
REFERENCES

Cooper, J., Moodley, M. and Reynell J. (1974). Intervention programmes for preschool children with delayed language development. A preliminary report. *British Journal of Disorders of Communication,* **9(2),** 81

Cooper J., Moodley, M. and Reynell J. (1978). *Helping Language Development.* (London: Edward Arnold)

Cooper, J., Moodley, M. and Reynell J. (1979). The developmental language programme: Results from a five year study. *British Journal of Disorders of Communication,* **14(2),** 57

Griffiths, Ruth (1970). *The Abilities of Young Children* (Child Development Research Centre)

Reynell, J. (1976). Early education of handicapped children. *Child: Care, Health and Development,* **2,** 305

Reynell, J. (1977). *Reynell Developmental Language Scales.* Revised Edition (NFER Publishing Company Ltd)

Reynell, J. (1979). Reynell–Zinkin Scales. *Developmental Scales for Young Visually Handicapped Children. Part 1: Mental Development*

Sonksen, P. M. (1977). The assessment needs of preschool children with handicaps of language development. *Child: Care, Health and Development,* **3,** 319

Wingfield, E. and Wingfield, A. (1970). Ladybird Picture Books (Loughborough: Wills and Hepworth Ltd)

APPENDIX II
READING LIST

I am indebted to the staff of the National Hospital College of Speech Sciences for help in compiling the following list of suggestions for further reading. The books are listed under three separate headings to aid selection.

LANGUAGE AND COMMUNICATION: GENERAL

Argyle, M. (1969). *Social Interaction.* (London: Methuen)

Clark, H. and Clark, E. (1977). *Psychology and Language.* (New York: Harcourt Brace Jovanovich)

Danziger, K. (1979). *Interpersonal Communication.* (Pergamon General Psychology Series) (Oxford: Pergamon Press)

Rick, D., and Wing, L. (1975). In: Lorna Wing (ed.) *Language, Communication and the Use of Symbols in Early Childhood Autism.* (Oxford: Pergamon Press)

Tanner, B. (ed.) (1976). *Language and Communication in General Practice.* (London: Hodder and Stoughton)

Vigotsky, L. S. (1962). *Thought and Language.* (Cambridge, Mass: MIT Press)

CHILD LANGUAGE, DEVELOPMENT AND LINGUISTICS

Cruttenden, A. (1979). *Speech in Infancy and Childhood* (Manchester: Manchester University Press)

Crystal, D. (1976). *Child Language, Learning and Linguistics* (London: Edward Arnold)

Dale, P. S. (1976). *Language Development, 2nd Edition*. (New York: Holt, Rinehart)

Herriot, P. (1971). *Language and Teaching: a Psychological View*. (London: Methuen)

Hopper, R. and Naremore, R. (1978). *Children's Speech. 2nd Edition*. (New York: Harper and Row)

Jeffree, D. and McConkey, R. (1976). *Let Me Speak*. (London: Souvenir Press)

Lee, L L. (1974). *Developmental Sentence Analysis*. (Chicago, Illinois: Northwestern University Press)

Lee, V. (1979). *Language Development*. (London: Croom Helm (OU Set Book))

Templin, M . C. (1957). *Certain Language Skills in Children* (Minneapolis: University of Minnesota Press)

Tough, J. (1976). *Listening to Children Talking*. (London: Ward Lock Educational)

CHILD LANGUAGE: DISABILITIES AND REMEDIATION

Berry, M. (1969). *Language Disorders of Children*. (New York: Appleton–Century–Crofts)

Berry, P. (ed.) (1976). *Language and Communication in the Mentally Handicapped* (London: Edward Arnold)

Clarke, A. D. B. and Lewis, M. M. (ed.) (1972). *Learning, Speech and Thought in the Mentally Retarded* (London: Butterworths)

Clezy, G. (1979). *Mother and Child Interaction*. (London: Edward Arnold)

Crystal D., Fletcher, P. and Garman, M. (1976). *The Grammatical Analysis of Language Disability* (London: Edward Arnold)

Darley, F. L. and Spriesterbach, D. C. (1978). *Diagnostic Methods in Speech Pathology. 2nd Edition*. (New York: Harper and Row)

Eisenson, J. (1952). *Aphasia in Children*. (New York: Harper and Row)

Gillham, W. (1979). *First Words Language Programme*. (London: George Allen and Beaconsfield Publishers)

Reading list

Ingram, D. (1976). *Phonological Disability in Children.* (London: Edward Arnold)

Irwin, J. V. and Marge, M. (1972). *Principles of Childhood Language Disabilities.* (New York: Appleton–Century–Crofts)

Karnes, M. (1968). *Helping Young Children Develop Language Skills.* (Reston, Virginia: The Council for Exceptional Children)

Lavalelli, C S. (1972). *Language Training in Early Childhood Education* (Chicago, Illinois: University of Illinois Press)

Lee L L., Koenigsknecht, R A. and Mulhern, S . T. (1975). *Interactive Language Development Teaching* (Chicago, Illinois: Northwestern University Press)

O'Connor, N. (1975). *Language, Cognitive Deficits and Retardation.* (London: Butterworths)

Royal National Institute for the Deaf (1976). *Methods of Communication Currently Used in Education of Deaf Children*

Rutter M. and Martin, J. A. M. (eds) (1972). *The Child with Delayed Speech. Clinics in Developmental Medicine No. 43.* (London: Spastics Society and Heinemann)

Wyke M. (1979). *Developmental Dysphasia.* (London: Academic Press)

Wells, C. (1971). *Cleft Palate and its Associated Speech Disorders.* (New York: McGraw–Hill)

APPENDIX III
SUGGESTED LIST OF
MATERIALS FOR ASSESSMENT

Real objects: Spoon, cup, hairbrush, toothbrush

Symbolic toys: Large doll or teddy, toy cup and child's brush

Doll's house size of doll, bed, blanket, chair, table.

Pictures: Clear coloured pictures of spoon, cup, hairbrush and toothbrush or any other pictures that can be matched to familiar objects, with objects and toys to match. Also some pictures that can be matched to gestures.

Toy box: A shoebox full of small toys including doll-play, cars, bricks and farm animals.

Index